8-WEEK WEIGHT LOSS PROGRAM

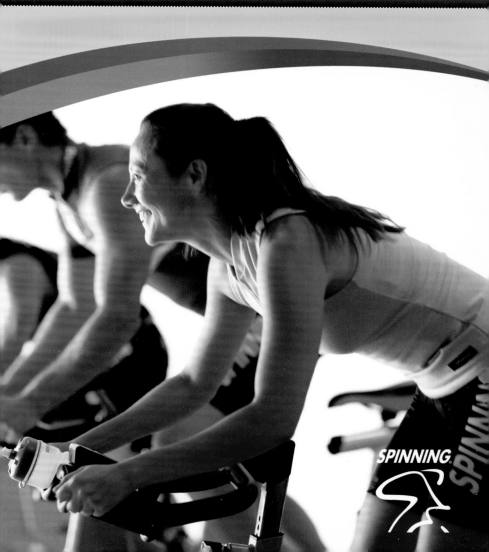

SPINNING

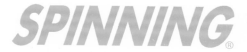

Welcome

Get ready to experience what just may be the healthiest eight weeks of your life. This program is not a diet—it's a plan you can live with. Whether you're new to the Spinning program or a longtime fan, you'll enjoy a new approach to getting fit and losing weight. The next eight weeks are going to be all about Healthy Habits, nutrition and plenty of calorie-burning Spinning rides! This manual explains everything you need to do to prepare, get started and reach your fitness and weight loss goals.

If you want to see what others are saying about the 8-Week Weight Loss Program, log on to community.spinning.com to visit our online forum! Join in the discussion by posting comments about your experiences, and get support from other participants around the world that are on the same 8-Week Weight Loss journey! *For users that do not already have a FREE Spinning account, go to www.spinning.com and "Create an Account." Then, use your spinning.com username and password to log onto community.spinning.com. Select the "Forums" tab and click on "8-Week Weight Loss Program" to participate in the forum.

Mad Dogg Athletics, Inc. 2111 Narcissus Ct. Venice, CA 90291

800.847.7746 310.823.7008 www.spinning.com

Contents

Read these sections prior to Week One.

Each week, read about that week's Healthy Habits and complete the exercises.

You can use these illustrated workouts to guide you through your exercise routine.

Mad Dogg Athletics
2111 Narcissus Court
Venice, California 90291

Tel 800.847.SPIN (7746) • www.spinning.com

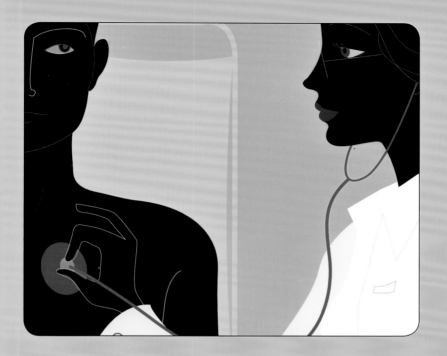

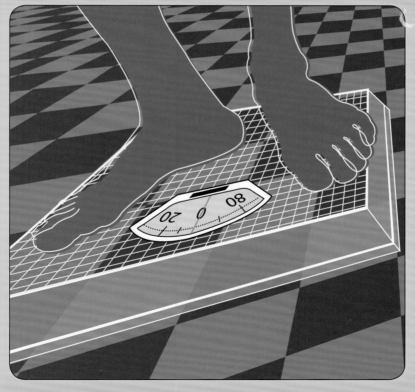

Welcome to the Spinning®
8-Week Weight Loss Program

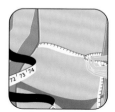

Congratulations and welcome! You are about to embark on The Spinning® 8-Week Weight Loss Program—a plan that will provide you with the tools, information and motivation you need to create Healthy Habits for fitness, wellness and weight loss.

This program is realistic and easy to follow—with a foundation based on sound nutrition principles and safe, energizing Spinning workouts. Whether you're a longtime fan of the Spinning program or brand new to indoor cycling, don't worry. The Spinning program is for everyone, and the Spinning 8-Week Weight Loss Program is for anyone who wants to take their health and fitness to a new level.

An Overview of the Program

Over the next eight weeks, you will experience a program that has been developed, tested and refined by fitness and nutrition experts, including Jennifer Ward, a Master Instructor for the Spinning program as well as registered dietician, certified lactation counselor and competitive cyclist. Jennifer has led successful weight loss programs with individuals ranging from competitive athletes to the overweight. This program is a culmination of her years of expertise, experience and dedication to health and fitness.

The 8-week program is set up like a "guided tour" that will take you through a series of exercises and trainings, all leading you to your new, healthier lifestyle. Along the way, you'll gain nutritional knowledge and heart rate training instructions. If the topics of nutrition or heart rate training sound intimidating, relax. It's easier than you think, and we'll take it one step at a time.

If you've had negative experiences with weight loss programs in the past, rest assured that this 8-week program places a positive "spin" on weight loss, it will help you change your eating and exercise patterns to elicit noticeable results that you can maintain indefinitely. Not only will you enjoy the way you look and feel after completing this program, but you will also enjoy the process through which you attain your results.

The Spinning® 8-Week Weight Loss Program is based on two fundamental elements. The first of these is exercise. You'll learn how to exercise at the appropriate intensity for your fitness level in order to burn fat and calories and improve your physical condition. The second is something we don't want to call "diet." Rather, it's a series of eight simple habits that you will incorporate two at a time to gradually improve your personal nutrition.

Before you begin the program, you'll read information about Spinning workouts, nutrition, and exercise. Taking the time to do this is essential, as the knowledge you gain will apply to every single week of the program—and, we hope, your life! Then you'll jump right in, using your new-found knowledge, week-by-week tips and your Spinning training to find a fitter you.

Before You Begin

Before you begin the program, there are a few topics to address. Take the time to read the following sections on Spinning program fundamentals, dieting, and lifestyle changes to help you understand the program, incorporate healthy habits and measure your improvements. You can refer back to these beginning sections as you progress through the course.

About the Spinning® Program

The Spinning program has become a global exercise and wellness phenomenon. Each day, thousands of certified Spinning Instructors help millions of people worldwide get into shape, have fun, train with purpose and enjoy a powerful mind-body connection.

Created in the 1980s by personal trainer and ultra-endurance athlete Johnny G, Spinning® is a unique indoor cycling training program. It brings the elements of athletic training to people of all fitness levels, but contrary to popular belief, Spinning is not just a "hard-core" fitness program for elite athletes. Instead, this high-energy exercise integrates music, camaraderie and visualization in a complete mind/body exercise program that is appropriate for participants of all ages and abilities. The Spinning® program uses the specially designed Spinner® stationary bike, heart rate training and a simple set of movements and hand positions to deliver personal empowerment and unparalleled fitness results. In fact, in just one 40-minute ride, riders will burn an average of 500 calories.

The following information will help you use a Spinner bike safely. There's also lots of setup and safety information available at www.spinning.com.

The Spinner® Bike

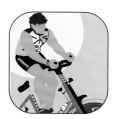

The patented Spinner bike is specially designed for the Spinning® program. The Spinner bike lets you change positions with ease and includes the following features to create an enjoyable, effective workout:

• A wide, padded seat to keep you comfortable and balanced. Adjust the seat horizontally and vertically to create a personalized fit.

• Adjustable handlebars featuring foam grips and a patented design that facilitates proper Spinning hand positions.

• An adjustable resistance knob to keep you in control of your ride. Simply twist the dial to add more or less resistance.

• A weighted flywheel to create a non-impact workout and facilitate a fluid pedal stroke.

Your Spinner bike uses a direct-drive fixed flywheel system that does not allow you to coast. To stop, decrease your speed gradually. **If you need to stop immediately, push down on the red resistance knob.**

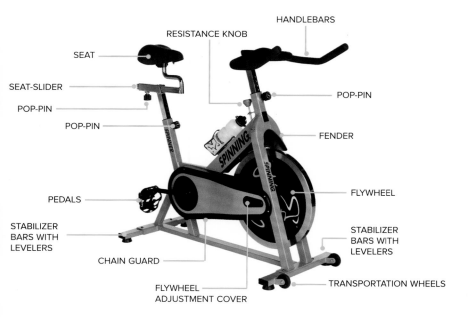

Safety in the Spinning® Program

Here are a few important safety guidelines to observe during your Spinning workout.

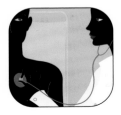

- Consult your physician before you begin an exercise program, especially if you're taking special medications, have been injured, had a recent surgery, or are pregnant.

- Before you ride, familiarize yourself with the bike and its operation. The Spinner® bike has a weighted flywheel and a fixed gear. To stop the pedals from moving, gradually reduce your leg speed. If you need to stop suddenly for any reason, push down on the resistance knob and keep your feet on the pedals until the flywheel comes to a stop.

- Always ride at your own pace, stay in control and focus on your form.

- If you begin to feel faint or dizzy, slowly stop pedaling and carefully dismount the bike.

Spinning® Program Fundamentals

> The Spinning program uses three hand positions and five core movements

Although individual workouts vary, the Spinning program is designed to encourage the fusion of mind and body in simulated rides that draw on visualization techniques, imagery and inspirational language. A gradual warm-up is followed by simulated terrain, including long flats, sprints, jumps and hill climbs using three hand positions and five core movements.

Hand Position 1 is used for warm-up, cool-down and recovery periods. Place the edges of your hands on the center part of the handlebars, maintaining a slight triangle between the fists and the elbows. Always keep the elbows and shoulders relaxed.

Hand Position 2 is used for running, jumping, sprinting and seated climbs. Place your hands outside the ring on the center of the handlebar. This position opens up the lungs to facilitate breathing and provides stability during out-of-the-saddle movements.

Hand Position 3 is only used for out-of-the-saddle climbs. Lightly grasp the ends of the handlebars, wrap your fingers and place your thumbs over the ends.

The Spinning program simulates real cycling terrain, conditions and techniques using five core movements that make real cycling sense.

At its core, the program consists of Seated Flats, Seated Climbs, Standing Climbs, Standing Flats, and Jumps that are all performed during varying ride conditions and terrain.

Seated Flat

The most basic movement in the Spinning® program, the Seated Flat, helps build a strong fitness base. Riders refer to the Seated Flat as "time in the saddle" because it develops physical strength, stamina and mental determination to weather long distances. During the Seated Flat, put your hands in Hand Position 1 or 2 and maintain a cadence (pedal speed) of 80-110 RPM.

Seated Climb

The Seated Climb is an efficient yet challenging movement that is performed with moderate to heavy resistance on the flywheel. During the Seated Climb, the buttocks naturally shift to the rear of the saddle, which increases the range of motion and allows the larger muscles of the body to assume the majority of the work. This movement challenges riders to develop a fluid pedal stroke, especially during periods of heavy resistance. To achieve this, ride in Hand Position 2 and maintain a consistent cadence of 60-80 RPM.

Standing Climb

The Standing Climb challenges you to ride out of the saddle with heavy resistance while in Hand Position 3. This movement involves the entire body in a realistic hill climb that adds power to the pedal stroke and strengthens and defines the leg muscles. Always keep your body weight centered over the pedals and advance into this movement gradually; this prevents unnecessary strain on the Achilles tendon, knees, hips and lower back. The slow and strenuous cadence of the Standing Climb should not exceed 60-80 RPM.

Standing Flat (Running)

The Standing Flat allows riders to take a break from the saddle and is also good preparation for Jumps. While pedaling with light to moderate resistance, stand up and begin running with light, rhythmic pedal strokes while your hands are in Hand Position 2. While running, shift your weight to the lower half of your body and center your weight over the pedals. The buttocks should just barely touch the nose of the saddle. Although your body will naturally shift from side to side with each downward stroke, always keep the hips level and facing forward. Maintain a cadence of 80-110 RPM.

Jumps

Before attempting Jumps, you will need a solid cycling fitness base and strong familiarity with the Spinning® program's basic seated and standing positions. Jumps are performed by moving from a seated to standing position at various intervals. This movement may be performed in two ways:

1. At a consistent pace, keeping the leg speed the same while moving in and out of the saddle with smooth, controlled movements.

2. With a burst of power, pedaling at a faster cadence to simulate breaking away from the pack in a race.

Jumps are challenging because they require riders to make smooth yet fast transitions in and out of the saddle at a steady cadence. To perform this movement, keep your weight centered in the lower body and lightly grasp the handlebars in Hand Position 2. Regardless of the intervals, your movements should be fluid and even; stop when fatigued or when form falters. Try to maintain a cadence of 80–110 RPM and always ride at your own pace.

Seated Flat	Seated Climb	Standing Climb	Standing Flat	Jumps
Hand Position 1 or 2 80-110 RPM	Hand Position 2 60-80 RPM	Hand Position 3 60-80 RPM	Hand Position 2 80-110 RPM	Hand Position 2 80-110 RPM

Spinner® Bike Setup

Proper bike setup and usage gives you a more comfortable ride and reduces your risk of injury.

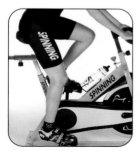

Seat Height

At the proper height, there should be a 25-35 degree bend in your knee at the bottom of a pedal stroke.

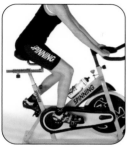

Fore/Aft Position

This refers to the seat's proximity to the handle-bars. When both pedals are level, your forward kneecap should be directly above the center of the pedal. Recheck the seat height again after making the fore/aft adjustment, as moving the seat forward or backward can have the same effect as moving it higher or lower.

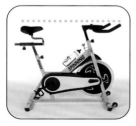

Handlebar Height

Position the handlebar at approximately the same height as your seat, or higher if you feel any dis-comfort in your back.

For more information
about bike setup, go to
www.spinning.com

Core Movements

These simple and effective core movements form the foundation of the Spinning program.

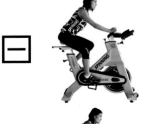

Seated Flat

Hand Position 1 or 2:
80-110 RPM
This basic movement builds strength and stamina.

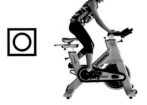

Standing Flat/Running

Hand Position 2
80-110 RPM
This movement is performed out-of-the-saddle using moderate resistance. "Running" develops core strength and increases endurance.

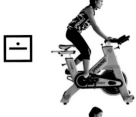

Jumps

Hand Position 2:
80-110 RPM
Jumps are performed by transitioning in and out of the saddle in smooth, controlled movements. Jumps develop overall strength, timing and balance by shifting from a seated to a standing position.

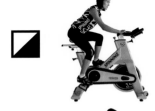

Seated Climb

Hand Position 2
60-80 RPM
This movement tones and strengthens the glutes and hamstrings.

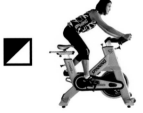

Standing Climb

Hand Position 3:
60-80 RPM
This out-of-the-saddle climb incorporates high resistance to strengthen and define the legs.

Advanced Movements

These advanced techniques are for riders who can perform core movements with good form and are ready for an increased challenge. Because these are advanced movements, they are only recommended for those who are experienced on the bike.

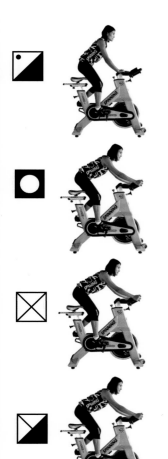

Running with Resistance
Hand Position 2
60-80 RPM
With moderate resistance, balance your weight over the center of the bike, grip lightly on the handlebars, relax your shoulders and hold your head in line with your spine.

Jumps on a Hill
Hand Positions 2 and 3
80-110 RPM
With heavy resistance, start out in a Seated Climb and transition to a Standing Climb, one hand at a time. Continue to transition between seated and standing.

Sprints
Hand Positions 2 and 3
80-110 RPM
With heavy resistance, explode out of the saddle into Hand Position 3. Once you "break" the gear, sit back in the saddle (Hand Position 2) and keep up the cadence for 20-30 seconds.

Sprints on a Hill
Hand Position 3
60-80 RPM
A Sprint on a Hill is similar to a Sprint, but with even more resistance to simulate the hill climbing. Explode out of the saddle (Hand Position 3) and push hard for 15-20 seconds.

Spinning® and Heart Rate Monitors

Why Use a Heart Rate Monitor?

You want your workout to count, right? Whether you exercise to burn fat and calories, feel energized or strengthen your cardiorespiratory system, your body needs to work at the right intensity...not too strenuous and not too light. Using a heart rate monitor is the best way to ensure that your Spinning workouts will deliver the results you want and will help you avoid weight loss plateaus, fatigue and injury.

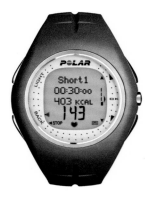

You may be thinking, "But why can't I just count my pulse or use rating of perceived exertion?" Those methods alone simply won't give you an accurate measure of your heart rate. Counting your pulse requires you to slow down your activity, which immediately drops your heart rate. RPE is a general gauge that can't really ensure that you're training in the right heart rate zone.

> **Need a heart rate monitor? Go to www.spinning.com or call 800. 847. 7746**

With a heart rate monitor, you can take your Spinning workouts to a whole new level. Use the chart below to train at the right intensity, measured in percent of max heart rate (MHR). You can estimate your MHR by subtracting your age from 220.

REASONS TO USE A HEART RATE MONITOR

1. To reach your fitness goals, you need to exercise at the right intensity.

2. Heart rate is a useful guide to tell you how difficult or easy your intensity is.

3. Using a heart rate monitor is the easiest and most accurate way to continuously measure your heart rate.

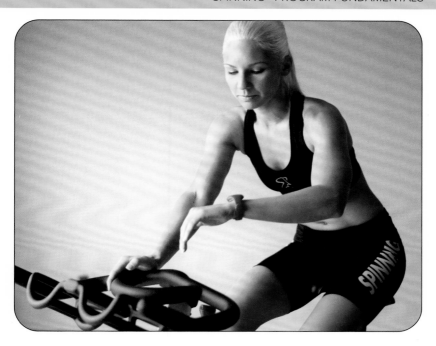

With a heart rate monitor, you can take your Spinning® workouts to a whole new level. Use the chart below to train at the right intensity, measured in percent of max heart rate (MHR). You can estimate your MHR by subtracting your age from 220.

Energy Zone™	Intensity Range	Purpose
Recovery	50% to 65% of MHR	Relaxation and energy accumulation.
Endurance	65% to 75% of MHR	Raises metabolism, burns fat, increases energy.
Strength	75% to 85% of MHR	Improves muscular endurance and mental stamina.
Interval	65% to 92% of MHR	Trains the heart to recover quickly from work effort.
Race Day	80% to 92% of MHR	Challenges the well conditioned exerciser.

Endurance Energy Zone™

The Endurance Energy Zone (EEZ) is the heart and soul of any successful training program and an integral part of the five Energy Zones of the Spinning® program.

The EEZ builds an aerobic foundation, increases aerobic capacity and improves cycling economy (meaning your body has to expend less energy at any given intensity). Endurance training should make up the largest percentage of your total training time. It is the foundation upon which you should build your fitness and performance goals. Whether you are a world-class athlete, a Spinning class regular or a beginning exerciser, most of your workout time should be spent in the Endurance zone.

Endurance Energy Zone Parameters
HEART RATE: 65-75% of max heart rate
RESISTANCE: Light to moderate
CADENCE: Maintain 80-110 RPM (perform a cadence check to determine leg speed)
FREQUENCY: 60-70% of total training time (two workouts/week if you exercise three times a week and three workouts/week if you exercise five times a week)

Benefits of Exercising in the Endurance Energy Zone
- Builds an aerobic base (foundation) which is critical for improving heart and lung capacity. Without a sufficient aerobic base, you'll lack the stamina necessary to exercise for long periods of time and to boost intensity.

- Increases your aerobic capacity, which affects the body's ability to generate fuel using oxygen, meaning you can work at a higher intensity but still utilize your more efficient aerobic "engine." High aerobic capacity also allows for faster recovery between workouts.

- Improves fat burning (metabolism) by increasing enzyme activity in the working muscles. This boosts your ability to use fat as an energy source. As you become more proficient training in the EEZ, you will burn more fat than you used to (which may be why you see your hips, thighs, arms and abdomen shrinking).

- Protects against heart attack and other cardiovascular diseases. The heart increases in size as a result of proper endurance training and the volume of blood it pumps with each stroke increases. This blood flow goes to nourish your working muscles. You may notice your resting heart rate decreasing as much as 1 beat/min. each week during your first month of aerobic base building. This is solid proof that your heart doesn't have to work as hard to pump the same amount of blood that it did before you started your endurance training.

- Improves oxygen consumption, which means that your body utilizes more oxygen during maximal exercise. The more oxygen your body can take in and put to "work," the more efficient you will be.

Interval Energy Zone™

If you want to take your training and conditioning to the next level, the Interval Energy Zone is an excellent way to get there.

The Interval Energy Zone (IEZ) is integral to any training program that's designed to enhance performance or competition. But interval training, or abruptly increasing and decreasing heart rate by manipulating the intensity of an activity, can also be beneficial for those who are simply looking for a way to enhance their level of fitness.

Interval Energy Zone Parameters

HEART RATE: There are three types of common intervals. Each one improves a specific energy system and relates to a certain heart rate range.

AEROBIC INTERVALS: performed at 50-80% of max heart rate (MHR)

AEROBIC/ANAEROBIC INTERVALS: performed at 65-92% of MHR

ANAEROBIC INTERVALS: Intensity is "all-out." No heart rate parameters are given because the duration of the interval is so short that the heart rate monitor cannot accurately reflect the actual work intensity. However, it's important to monitor the recovery portion of this intense interval by dropping your heart rate in 2-5 minutes after going anaerobic.

WORK-TO-REST RATIOS:
- Aerobic = 4-15 minutes of work effort followed by 15-30 seconds of recovery
- Aerobic/Anaerobic = 30 seconds to 10 minutes of work effort followed by an equal amount of recovery.
- Anaerobic = 5-20 seconds of work followed by two to five minutes of recovery

CADENCE: 80-110 RPM in the flats and 60-80 RPM in the hills

FREQUENCY: 5-10% of total training time should be spent in the IEZ (approx. once a week).

Remember, you should spend at least two months training in the Endurance EZ to build an effective aerobic base (foundation) before completing an Internal EZ ride. Aerobic base building is critical in developing improvements in the heart and lungs and in developing the body's ability to store and trans-port fuel and produce energy. Neglect this foundation, and you will lack stamina for the more intense training demands required during the IEZ.

Benefits of Exercising in the Interval Energy Zone

• Interval training can increase aerobic and anaerobic capacity. By repeatedly exposing active muscles to high-intensity exercise, you improve their resistance to fatigue. As a result, riders will be able to sustain a given exercise intensity for a longer period of time, thus increasing their endurance.

• Interval training teaches the body to recover quickly after a challenging work bout. This is important to overall fitness because the primary stimulus for cardiovascular improvement occurs during the recovery phase of the interval.

Recovery Energy Zone™

The "easy" EZ is really one of the most difficult to master. Are you savvy enough to know when—and how—to use it?

The Recovery Energy Zone (REZ) is a particularly important part of the Spinning® program, especially now that enthusiasts are training harder and longer than ever before. The Spinning program is comprised of five Energy Zones: Recovery, Endurance, Strength, Interval and Race Day. Without the REZ, the big picture—a balanced fitness program—is incomplete. The REZ helps restore muscles, ligaments, tendons and other parts of the body after strenuous exercise; it actually increases your work capacity and improves performance. Without sufficient recovery, it's impossible to make significant fitness gains. Neglecting the recovery component of training can result in lowered performance, illness and/or injury.

Recovery Energy Zone Parameters
HEART RATE: 50-65% of age predicted maximum heart rate (MHR)
RESISTANCE: Light
CADENCE: 80-110 RPM
FREQUENCY: Participants taking five to seven Spinning classes per week should schedule one recovery class per week. Elite athletes who train twice a day need two or more days of recovery, depending on the time of year and intensity of training.

Benefits of Exercising in the Recovery Energy Zone
• The Recovery Energy Zone increases the ability of muscular and cardiovascular systems to recover from high-intensity training sessions and is referred to as "active recovery," as opposed to "passive recovery," which would include getting a massage, taking a warm bath or sitting on the couch with the remote. Certainly, there's a time and place for both active and passive recovery—both are important. However, active recovery has been proven to be more effective in removing excess lactic acid from the muscles compared to passive recovery.

• A hard training session (Interval, Race Day and even Strength) depletes blood glucose from your system and fatigues the central nervous system (CNS). Recovery training sessions will stimulate and promote blood circulation. It's not the high-intensity training sessions that make you stronger; it's the recovery process that gives your body time to process those training adaptations. Without the overload, your body is not stimulated to improve, and without rest, the body gets overstressed and becomes susceptible to illness and injury. Finally, the Recovery Energy Zone increases feelings of relaxation, balance and well-being and is considered an active form of meditation. Use that time to visualize positive images that will contribute to your success.

Strength Energy Zone™

The Strength Energy Zone (SEZ) is a unique training experience and an integral part of the five Energy Zones that make up the Spinning® program. This Energy Zone builds your muscular strength, endurance and cardiovascular system. The SEZ trains the ligaments and tendons of the legs to handle high-intensity training and improves power and climbing ability.

Strength Energy Zone Parameters
HEART RATE: Program your heart rate monitor for 75-85% of max heart rate.
RESISTANCE: Constant resistance (moderate to heavy load) on the legs during the work portion of the class. You will be on a hill for the entire work portion.
CADENCE: 60-80 RPM
FREQUENCY: Depending on your goals, you must first build an aerobic base before you participate in a SEZ class. Performing a SEZ class too early in your training can lead to injury. Aim for no more than two strength classes per week.

Benefits of Exercising in the Strength Energy Zone

• The SEZ straddles the aerobic and anaerobic system in the body, so you have options when you train in this Energy Zone. When riding in the lower half of the SEZ (75-80% MHR), you are still in your aerobic zone, developing your fat-burning system, strengthening your immune system and creating more energy producing sites in your muscles.

• When riding in the upper half of the SEZ (80-85% MHR) you are in your anaerobic zone, learning how to tolerate lactic acid and build the cardiovascular ability to handle a slightly uncomfortable pace for a long duration of time. You can use the entire range of 75-85% MHR in this class to acquire the mental and physical benefits of both aerobic and anaerobic training.

• From a mental training standpoint, the SEZ will help you understand how to relax and focus while working. You will learn how to turn adversity (the hill or lactic acid build-up) into an opportunity (lactate tolerance or overcoming obstacles). Your psychological intensity will increase as you push through increased intensities and   changes in workloads. As you overcome the challenge of climbing the hill, your self-confidence will also increase.

• Recovery is critical after a SEZ class, due to the constant resistance that you're applying and the muscular soreness that is created. We recommend you take 48-72 hours off between SEZ classes. The body needs time to adapt to the form of training stress that is applied to the muscles. Just as you wouldn't train your biceps muscles   every day, you wouldn't train your heart and leg muscles the same way every day.

Race Day Energy Zone™

Race Day is your chance to test yourself, to put everything you've learned through all those weeks of training on the table. Are you up for the challenge?

The Race Day Energy Zone (RDEZ) is a celebration, an opportunity to apply the training you've been practicing toward a peak performance effort. This means that you should take every measure to ensure that you are both physically and mentally ready for such a challenge. The RDEZ is not to be taken lightly; it requires complete focus, dedication and determination. A Race Day ride can help you effectively measure your goal setting as it relates to your Spinning®/cycling training plan.

Race Day Energy Zone Parameters

HEART RATE: 80-92% of MHR

RESISTANCE: Resistance can range from intense climbs to challenging flats. The key to remember is that the rider who pushes the biggest gear with an aggressive leg speed (80-110 RPM) is the rider who will clock the fastest time. You will not clock the fastest time, burn the most calories, become stronger as an athlete or sculpt and define your leg muscles by using low resistance and turning the flywheel as fast as you can. The bottom line: resistance training first, speed later.

CADENCE: 80-110 RPM

FREQUENCY: Race Day can be used as a monthly test to determine whether your training plan is making you more fit. It will allow you to have a better understanding of your HR potential and create a wider paradigm for training.

Benefits of Exercising in the Race Day Energy Zone

- Race Day training challenges your body to work at higher heart rates, close to and above your anaerobic threshold (AT). Anaerobic threshold marks the point where lactate accumulates in the bloodstream faster than it can be removed. Purposely taking your body to this point and beyond forces it to adapt to greater concentrations of lactic acid, which will dramatically improve your AT.

- These training sessions engage the muscle fibers and train them to go faster, to have more available energy and to recover more quickly after exhausting training.

- A race is not a place to work on weaknesses; however there is much to learn from each racing experience. Participation in each Race Day session will help you gauge your progress, realize your potential and highlight any weaknesses in your training plan.

Terminology

Throughout this program, you may come across some words or terms that are unfamiliar to you, or words that you've heard, but don't know the definitions of. The following is a list of terms that you'll need to understand to get the most out of this program.

Aerobic Exercise: In aerobic exercise, the body uses stored fat and carbohydrates for energy. At 70-80% of your maximum heart rate, 50% of the calories you burn are from fat and the other 50% are carbohydrates. This is excellent for increasing the number and size of your blood vessels, increasing your vital capacity and respiratory rates and achieving increases in pulmonary ventilation and arterial venous oxygen.

Anaerobic Exercise: Anaerobic exercise can be used to build your heart/lung capacity and endurance. In it, the body burns more calories (but mostly from carbohydrates rather than fat). At 80-90% of your maximum heart rate, 15% of the calories you burn are from fat, and 85% are carbohydrates. This improves your VO2 max (the highest amount of oxygen one can consume during exercise) and thus imrproves your heart/lung system and gives you a higher lactate tolerance ability, which means your endurance will improve and you'll be better equipped to fight fatigue.

Anaerobic Threshold: The transition phase between aerobic and anaerobic exercise. Good training will increase AT by teaching the muscles to use oxygen more efficiently so that less lactic acid is produced. Also known as "lactate threshold."

Basal Metabolic Rate: (BMR) is the number of calories your body burns at rest to maintain normal body functions. It changes with age, weight, height, gender, diet and exercise habits.

Bioelectrical Impedance Analysis: A method of estimating the amount of body weight that is fat and nonfat. Nonfat weight comes from bone, muscle, body water, organs, and other body tissues. BIA works by measuring how difficult it is for a harmless electrical current to move through the body. The more fat a person has, the harder it is for electricity to flow through the body. The less fat a person has, the easier it is for electricity to flow through the body. By measuring the flow of electricity, one can estimate body fat percentage.

Body Composition: The percentage of body fat to lean body mass.

Body Mass Index: A measure of mass that is calculated as weight in kilograms divided by height in meters squared.

Calorie Deficit: When the number of calories that one burns in a day exceeds the number of calories eaten in a day.

Carbohydrate: Carbohydrates are organic compounds that consist of carbon, hydrogen and oxygen. They vary from simple sugars to very complex polysaccharides. Carbohydrates provide 4 calories per gram. Plants manufacture and store carbohydrates as their chief source of energy. The glucose synthesized in the leaves of plants is used as the basis for more complex forms of carbohydrates. Classification of carbohydrates relates to their structural core of simple sugars (saccharides). Principal monosaccharides that occur in food are glucose and fructose. Three common disaccharides are sucrose, maltose and lactose. Polysaccharides of interest in nutrition include starch, dextrin, glycogen and cellulose.

Diabetic Exchange Lists: The dietary exchange system is a collaborative creation of the American Dietetic Association and the American Diabetes Association. In simplest terms, exchanges are an effort to make menu choices easier for people with diabetes and other special dietary needs.

Fat: A soft, greasy substance occurring in organic tissue and consisting of a mixture of lipids, which contain 9 calories per gram.

Glycemic Index: A ranking of foods based on their immediate effect on blood sugar levels. The glycemic index measures how much your blood sugar increases over a period of two or three hours after a meal (in creating this scale, the portion sizes of all foods contained 50 grams of carbohydrate).

Glycemic Load: The glycemic load of a food is calculated by multiplying the glycemic index by the amount of carbohydrate (in grams) provided by a food and dividing the total by 100. In essence, each unit of the glycemic load represents the equivalent blood glucose-raising effect of 1 gram of pure glucose or white bread. The concept of glycemic load was developed by scientists to simultaneously describe the quality (glycemic index) and quantity of carbohydrates in a meal or diet.

Glycogen: Glycogen is a large, complex carbohydrate molecule that is produced from glucose in the liver and muscles when blood sugar levels are high. Glycogen is broken down into lactic acid when it is used as an energy source in the liver or muscles.

Hydrogenation: Hydrogenation is the process of forcing hydrogen atoms into the holes of unsaturated fatty acids and is usually used to increase the shelf life of processed foods. These types of fats are not easily processed by the body, making weight loss difficult and sometimes negatively affecting health. Scientists have barely scratched the surface of studying changes induced in fats and oils by partial hydrogenation. The end result is many of these altered substances are toxic to our systems.

MHR: Maximum Heart Rate.

Obesity: The condition of being significantly overweight, usually defined as 30 percent or more over ideal body weight. Obesity puts a strain on the heart and can increase the chance of developing high blood pressure and diabetes.

Protein: A large, complex molecule composed of amino acids. The sequence of the amino acids, and thus the function of the protein, is determined by the sequence of the base pairs in the gene that encodes it. Proteins are essential to the structure, function, and regulation of the body. Examples are hormones, enzymes, and antibodies. Each gram of protein provides 4 calories per gram of usable energy.

> Benefits of resistance training include increased muscle mass, improved posture, increased fat-burning potential and reduced risk of injuries.

Resistance Training: Fitness training involves opposing force or resistance on the body. Resistance can come in various forms such as free weights, machines, elastic tubing, medicine balls or even your own body weight (crunches, for example). Some of the primary benefits of resistance training include increased muscle mass, improved posture, increased fat-burning potential, increased strength, increased endurance, increased stability, increased bone density, reduced risk of diseases (such as arthritis, heart disease and diabetes) and reduced risk of injuries.

Skin Caliper Test: A body composition method that uses calipers (or a gauge) to measure skin fold thicknesses. Skin fold thickness measurements are usually taken from at least three different sites.

Whole grains: Whole grains are high in fiber (whole wheat has five times the fiber of refined wheat). Unlike refined grains, whole grains are antioxidant-rich, tumor suppressors, cholesterol reducers, insulin regulators, antithrombotic agents, phytoestrogens and rich in vitamin E, folic acid, zinc, selenium and magnesium.

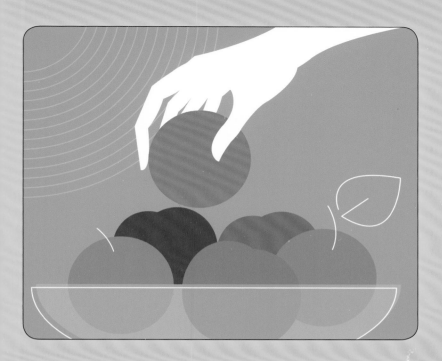

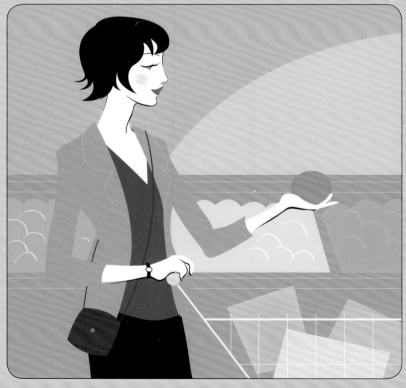

Diet is a Four-Letter Word

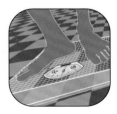

Now that you understand a little more about the Spinning® program, let's dive into the concept of dieting. What is the real definition of the word diet? How do people perceive it? How can you change this concept into something that is enjoyable and effective? It is hard to live in America and not notice the fact that such a large percentage of the population struggles with their weight. Most people believe that the solution to this problem is to go on a diet—as indicated by the billions of dollars that are poured into weight loss plans every year. Unfortunately, adult obesity has increased by 60 percent since 1991, meaning that not only has the media's push to diet failed to fix the problem, but as noted by the article excerpt below, it may have ignited it.

The decision to restrict one's eating, or diet, is usually made in the context of an attempt at self-improvement. For several decades, the North American cultural ethos has been that most of us are too fat (whether this is objectively true or not), and the solution was for the majority of people, especially women, to restrain their eating and follow weight loss diets. People dieted in the expectation that this would help them achieve enhanced health, appearance and feelings of well-being. It has become clear, however, that this "solution" did not solve the problem. In fact, given the increase in obesity in the Western world since the 1970s, when the dieting ethic began to dominate societal consciousness, it could be argued that the emphasis on dieting may have contributed to the increase in overweight. Arguments about the efficacy of dieting aside, however, what are the psychological ramifications of dieting or food restriction?

Janet Polivy, Ph.D.
"Psychological Consequences of Food Restriction"
The Journal of the American Dietetic Association, June 1996

The Results of Severe Food Restriction

Most people associate diet with food restriction. While it's true that through this program you will learn to avoid certain unhealthy foods and decrease your portion sizes, we need to be clear that severe food restriction will do more harm than good. There is a classic psychological study of food restriction that provides compelling data.

In the study, normal-weight (presumably non-dieting) men were asked to restrict their eating for 6 months to lose 25% of their initial body weight so that the effects of starvation could be studied. The men were fed only 75% of their normal intake and when they stopped losing weight, their food was further restricted until they got down to approximately 76% of initial body weight. These subjects were carefully observed over several months, and some interesting psychological reactions were noted. One change was that subjects became increasingly focused on food; they collected recipes, hung pinup pictures of food, and changed career plans to food-related activities such as becoming a chef. They also grew increasingly upset and irritable, fighting with each other and their girlfriends. The men appeared apathetic and lethargic and seemed to lose interest in sex (replacing pictures of women with their food pinups!). In some respects, the most striking changes occurred during the semi-starvation period and after weight was restored to normal and the study had ended. When the men were subsequently allowed to eat as much as they wanted, these previously normal, healthy eaters began to gorge themselves when attractive foods were available. Moreover, they report-ed feeling out of control of their eating and obsessed with food; some even stole food or gum. Food restriction actually appeared to produce binge eating in previously normal eaters.

Janet Polivy, Ph.D.
"Psychological Consequences of Food Restriction"
The Journal of the American Dietetic Association, June 1996

Does this mean that if you try to "diet," you are doomed to become obsessed with food, suffer from relationship problems, fluctuate in weight and experience erratic eating behavior? No, but you may need to rethink your definition of the word diet and how to go about creating permanent weight loss.

Exercise: Write down words, phrases and descriptions that come to mind when you think of the word diet.

_____

_____

_____

_____

_____

_____

_____

_____

What did you come up with? Were your answers similar to the ones listed below?

- Being hungry all of the time
- Not being able to eat when you want
- Not eating what you want
- Not eating as much as you want
- Eating only foods that taste bad
- Eliminating food groups
- Something that you do for a short period of time
- Not eating fat
- Not eating carbohydrates or sugar

Most of these phrases are negative and describe an unpleasant experience. Why would you want to pursue something that makes you miserable? On the off chance that putting yourself through misery does cause weight loss, how are you going to maintain those results if you did not enjoy what you did to get them?

> Exercise: List words, phrases and action steps that come to mind when you think of increasing fitness and improving body composition.

What were your answers this time? Perhaps you came up with answers similar to the ones listed below.

- Exercising more consistently
- Eating healthier
- Lifting weights
- Feeling better

- Eating less
- Eating less fat
- Avoiding junk food

The answers to the second exercise are more positive, and the few restrictions that come up seem more manageable—perhaps manageable enough that they could be maintained long-term.

The word diet is a term that was intended to define an individual's eating pattern. We're all on a "diet" because we all choose food or a calorie source to keep our bodies running. Instead, the term diet has come to mean restricting calories or doing crazy things to lose a few pounds. Once people reach their goals, they go off their diets and their plan is to somehow "maintain" their weight by not doing any of the things that they did to lose it.

Exercising until you drop 20 pounds will not cause permanent change. Neither will eliminating carbohydrates or alcohol until you lose *another* 10 pounds.

> Our bodies are very good at telling us what we need. We just need to get better at listening to them.

Changing into a person who exercises 45 minutes per day, 5 days per week *will* cause permanent change. Changing into a person who eats dessert twice per week instead of twice per day will also cause permanent change. Changing from a person who used to "binge-eat" at night in front of the television into someone who no longer snacks after dinner will likewise create permanent change.

You should not want to follow this program just to lose weight. In the Spinning® 8-Week Weight Loss Program, you are not going to count calories. This program is one that teaches you how to follow healthy eating guidelines, increase your activity and exercise at appropriate intensity levels. In place of counting calories, you will focus on learning how to pay attention to and follow your hunger and satiety signals. Our bodies are very good at telling us what we need, we just need to get better at listening to them. By making healthy changes and tracking them, you will find that over time they become habits, and you will naturally be able to continue them once you complete the program.

Breaking Down Barriers for Lifestyle Change

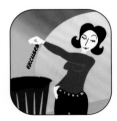

To say that you want something means nothing unless you are ready to take action and do something about it. You cannot just wish your way into better fitness. Nobody can. If some people put as much effort into getting fit and eating healthier as they do into making excuses, they would have been fit a long time ago. Start creating solutions rather than more excuses.

Excuse #1: "I don't have time to exercise."

Solution: It's true. It's difficult for many of us to find the time to exercise. But if you schedule it in as a priority, you'll be more successful. Every Sunday, decide on your Spinning workouts or activity times for the upcoming week and write those "appointments" into your day planner.

Excuse #2: "I have bad genes."

Solution: You can only compare you to you. While "genes" are often blamed for one's weight, more often than not one generation in a family passes bad eating and activity patterns to the next generation. Admittedly, you probably do not have control over your height, frame size, where you gain weight and the area from which you lose weight. However, this program is about improving yourself. No matter what gene cards you were dealt, changing your eating habits and increasing your activity levels will result in a healthier you.

Excuse #3: "I only eat bad food once in a while."

Solution: You may have eaten a hot dog for the first time in months on Wednesday; on Thursday you ate cheesecake for the first time in a year, on Friday you went to a party and had four mixed drinks, but that was okay because you hadn't had a drink for six months. The list could go on. In the example above, the individual splurged on some high-calorie foods that they had denied themselves for quite some time. Yet, upon further examination, they consistently made choices in food that were bound to impede their success. Keeping a food log can be helpful in sorting out whether or not you are inhibiting your success. If you cannot resist high-calorie treats, then at least choose small portion sizes.

> **If you cannot resist high-calorie treats, then at least choose small portion sizes.**

Excuse #4: "I am exercising as much as I can and nothing is happening."

Solution: Track what you are doing for exercise. Be as detailed as possible. Be honest. Include duration, intensity, frequency and distance covered. Many people discover that they are not doing as much as they think they are. On the other hand, if you are exercising 2 hours per week and not finding a difference, then adding 30 minutes per week may be the catalyst you need to induce a change.

Excuse #5: "I already eat all fat-free foods."

Solution: Whatever changes you make in your diet, if weight loss is your goal, you need to do it in a way that creates a calorie deficit. If you reduce your fat intake by cutting out butter and mayonnaise (for example), as long as you do not replace it with a substitute that is equal or greater in calories, you will probably experience some success. If you buy a package of fat-free cookies to replace the original version and proceed to eat twice the serving size, don't be surprised when the scale doesn't budge.

Shrinking Myths

The diet industry is always looking for opportunities to make more money. There is tremendous pressure to create new "twists" or unlock special 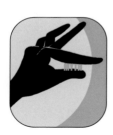 "secrets" that portray weight loss as an effortless process. Of course, most of these "twists and revelations" are outright lies. Weight loss can occur, but not for the reasons you are told. Furthermore, weight loss takes work. It does not have to be painful, but it will take time. It takes both thought and determination to retrain yourself on how to eat healthfully and how to find an exercise volume that works for you. Here are a few of the myths that we would like to debunk:

Myth #1: There are no bad or good foods as long as you eat everything in moderation.

According to the American Dietetic Association "all foods can fit" and "there are no good or bad foods as long as you eat them in moderation." However, since many of us choose foods for psychological reasons, we cannot underestimate the draw toward certain "comfort foods." If you find that you are choosing foods for the wrong reasons, or choosing foods that are higher in calories or fat more frequently than you choose healthy foods, then you may want to consider the following four points:

1. Allow yourself to eat something "bad." By trying to eliminate a food from your diet, you may find that you create an obsession with that food. Giving yourself permission to eat it may be enough to make eating that food in moderation a possibility.

2. Avoid it. There are some foods that are just hard to eat in controlled portions. Sometimes, not having any is better than having a little bit when "a little bit" always turns into "way too much." There is a saying "out of sight, out of mind." If you do not see it or it is not available, then you will adapt and learn not to miss it.

3. Include the food in your diet, but set limits on your portion sizes. For example, eating a full pint of ice cream would be counterproductive to losing weight, but on the other hand, a 1/2 cup might be okay. Think about it. If you want more of that food, you can have it again another day.

4. Find a healthier substitute for the food (but be mindful of the portion size). Save calories by using balsamic vinegar in place of creamy ranch salad dressing. If you choose a "fat-free" version of a food in place of the original version, make sure that there is a difference in calories between the two products and that you monitor the portion size. In many cases, manufacturers add so much sugar to fat-free foods that they end up being the same number of calories as their fat-containing versions!

Myth #2: All carbohydrates cause your body to store fat. To lose weight, you need to eliminate most of them from your diet.
Many high protein diet programs state that the restriction of carbohydrates without attention to calories is all that it takes for weight loss success. People who buy into these programs love them, because they enjoy eating high-protein, high-fat foods that they may have been previously eliminating for weight loss. They typically do not realize that they are restricting calories.

The thought that the public would go so far as to think that they need to restrict their intake of fruit, milk, whole grains and starchy vegetables should cause concern for the following reasons:

• It is possible to greatly diminish one's carbohydrate stores during a single workout, while it is impossible to do the same for fat and protein. Therefore, it makes sense that we would need to eat a greater volume of carbohydrates in comparison to fat and protein. Think about it. How far would you be able to go in your car if you changed the oil every week, but only filled the tank with gas once per month? Whether you are considering cars or humans, the fuel that is depleted most rapidly needs to be replaced most frequently.

• Our bodies burn fat more efficiently in the presence of carbohydrates. The body is less likely to break down muscle for energy when it is getting an adequate supply of carbohydrates.

Carbohydrates are stored in the liver and muscles as glycogen. The body stores an additional three parts of water for every one part of carbohydrate that is stored in the body in the form of glycogen. Restricting carbohydrates is exciting at first for most people because the number on the scale will initially drop rapidly due to water loss rather than fat loss or a true change in body composition. Additionally, decreased carbohydrate stores will lead to decreased performance during exercise sessions.

> **All individuals following The Spinning® 8-Week Weight Loss Program should consume no less than 45% of their calories from carbohydrate.**

"Breaking down" muscle is counter-productive to anyone who would like to improve body composition. A pound of muscle weighs the same as a pound of fat. However, a pound of muscle will increase the number of calories your body burns in a day and it takes up a much smaller volume than a pound of fat. If you diet improperly and lose muscle, then you may find it increasingly difficult to maintain or continue to lose weight.

- Eliminating whole grains, fruits and vegetables (even starchy vegetables) is extremely counterproductive to improving health and losing weight. Fruits and vegetables contain fiber, which promotes intestinal health, improves cholesterol levels and decreases the number of calories that the body absorbs. Additionally, whole grain foods, fruits and vegetables contain over 200,000 compounds called phytonutrients. Phytonutrients are compounds that work to prevent cancer and many other types of common diseases. There are just too many health benefits to even consider elimination or restriction of these foods in pursuit of weight loss.

While it is true that most people consume too much sugar, most of the sugar you should reduce is the refined white sugar that is added to many of the sweet treats and fat-free foods that are often touted as being "healthier." You can healthfully reduce your caloric intake by choosing foods that contain lower amounts of sugar and selecting products that do not have added sugar. In an attempt to reduce sugar, we do not recommend that you replace sugar with artificial sweeteners! Artificial sweeteners can stimulate hunger and have other negative side effects. When it comes to fruit, it is better to eat whole fruit than to drink juice. Whole fruit takes longer to eat, and provides more satiety and fiber.

Sometimes, carbohydrates are consumed in the form of refined white flour. Refined flour products have been stripped of many of their vitamins, minerals and fiber. As a result, they are digested quickly and may not satiate for long. While it is not necessary to completely eliminate all refined flours from your diet, it does make a lot of sense to read the ingredient labels on packages. If a product lists the word "whole" before the type of flour (e.g., whole wheat flour, whole oat flour, whole rye flour), then that food will usually contain more fiber, vitamins and minerals and provide a steadier source of energy. Whenever possible, you should choose a whole grain product that does not have added sugars instead of a refined flour product.

Many low-carbohydrate diet programs also use a scale called the "glycemic index." The glycemic index is a scale that is used to determine how quickly a food will cause a rise in blood sugar levels. All too often, this scale is taken too literally. For example, several different low-carbo-hydrate programs suggest that followers avoid carrots because they may have a high glycemic index. The glycemic index is highly flawed because each food is tested individually, when in reality, most people eat a few different foods at the same time. Secondly, the volume of food that is eaten when the glycemic index is tested is not necessarily comparable to the portion size that an individual eats in one sitting. Thirdly, different individuals will have different reactions to the same food. Therefore, it is safe to say that no one has a weight problem because they eat too many carrots! It makes no sense to eliminate a food that is natural, low in calories, high in fiber and contains cancer-fighting properties.

All individuals following the Spinning® 8-Week Weight Loss Program should consume no less than 45 percent of their calories from carbohy-drate, because of how many carbohydrates they will burn for fuel while exercising.

If you want to make the right decisions about food, you need to examine the whole picture, not just one tiny aspect of it.

Myth #3: Consuming the right ratio of fat, protein and carbohydrate will put your body into a "fat-burning zone."

There is no single rule you can follow every time you eat. Following a plan that encourages eating foods in a specific ratio may improve overall diet, but the fact remains that weight loss occurs primarily due to a calo-rie deficit (the same goes for low carbohydrate diets). Consuming carbohydrates with fat and protein can slow digestion and keep an individual satisfied longer, so there is some merit to combining carbohydrate-containing foods with fat and protein. On the con-trary, there are certain times when you might not want to consume fat and pro-tein. Carbohydrates are utilized the most quickly during exercise sessions. But eating fat and protein immediately before or after exercise could cause discomfort. Additionally, always

> There is no single way to eat all the time.

having to measure amounts of food so that specific ratios of carbohy-drate, fat and protein are achieved can be very tedious.

Myth #4: Skipping meals is a great way to save calories and lose weight.

Truth: Skipping meals is a great way to encourage your body to burn calories at a slower rate and make it more difficult for you to choose healthy foods and consume reasonable portion sizes when you finally do eat. When you skip breakfast, you may slow the rate that your body burns calories by as much as 40 percent! That means an individual with a basal metabolic rate (the number of calories burned per day excluding all activity) of 1,200 calories a day may drop that rate to 720 calories per day just by skipping breakfast! While the most significant *negative* effects occur when skipping breakfast, skipping other meals or not having healthy snacks when necessary can further impede weight loss by creat-ing an obsession with food.

You should also know that sugar cravings are most often caused by going too long without eating. Not starving yourself is one of the most effective ways to cure a sugar addiction!

Myth #5: Being very strict so that you lose a lot of weight and get motivated is a good way to start a diet.

You are only capable of losing about 1 pound of fat per week. If you have large amounts of weight to lose then you may find that your weight

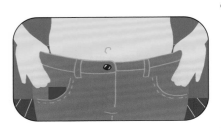

drops by more than a pound per week, but in most cases, only a pound of it is fat. In addition, being overly restrictive, even if it is for just a couple weeks at the beginning of a diet, makes it increasingly difficult to avoid overindulging or overcompen-sating later on. The Spinning® 8-Week Weight Loss Program is about making gradual, maintainable changes. Starting a program with extreme exercise and/or calorie-restriction will not support your overall goal.

Again, it is much easier to maintain weight loss when you make changes that you are able to continue long-term. If you lose weight ini-tially due to extreme exercise or extreme calorie restriction, there will come a time when you can no longer manage those extremes.

Myth #6: You need to lose a lot of weight to look different and be healthier.

Modest weight loss, especially when it is achieved through healthy eating and exercise, can dramatically change appearance and cause significant improvements in health (such as lower cholesterol and decreased blood pressure). As stated earlier, there is a limit to how much fat you can lose per week, but the rate of change in tape measurements and/or body composition can be dramatic in a relatively short period of time.

In reality, fitness and body composition improvement is a much better way of tracking progress. Most people care the most about weight, so that is why The Spinning 8-Week Weight Loss Program tracks it. But in all honesty, would you care if you didn't lose weight, but were able to drop two sizes? By the end of the eight weeks you will be the most excited about how you look and feel. Weight loss will just be an added bonus.

Weight Loss 101

Weight loss can occur for the following reasons:

1. Increasing your energy output by increasing:
   - Your volume of activity
   - The intensity of activity
   - The frequency of activity
   - Your muscle mass (thereby increasing the rate that your body burns calories)

2. Decreasing your caloric intake by eating:
   - Smaller portions
   - Fewer calories
   - Lower calorie foods
   - Less frequently in some cases
   - More frequently in some cases
   - More fiber (fiber can decrease the number of calories your body absorbs and can provide satiety)

3. Increasing the rate that your body burns calories by:
   - Increasing muscle mass through resistance training
   - Allowing adequate recovery between training sessions
   - Eating at least 45% of your calories from carbohydrate
   - Eating breakfast
   - Not allowing yourself to reach the point of "starvation"

Weight loss is most commonly approached by counting calories and trying to consume a specific amount each day. For example, consider individuals who decide to follow a 1,600-calorie diet. Most of the time, they strive to stick to that calorie intake regardless of how their day went. If they have a lazy Saturday and stay in bed for half the day and watch television for the other half, they eat 1,600 calories. The next day, they participate in a 2-hour Spinning® journey and eat 1,600 calories. Do you see the problem with this? On the Saturday that they did nothing, they may have eaten more than they needed. On the following day when they did the Spinning ride, they were probably starving! It is just as harmful to not eat when you are truly hungry as it is to eat when you are not hungry. Following a specific daily-calorie diet should be a last resort. If you like to count calories, you can find hundreds of different plans by doing a search on the Internet. The Spinning® 8-Week Weight Loss Program is about learning how to use your hunger and satiety signals as a guide and to learn good nutrition by following Healthy Habits.

> It is just as harmful to not eat when you are truly hungry as it is to eat when you are not hungry.

Nutrition 101: Food Groups

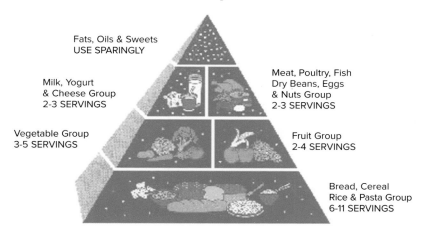

Fats, Oils & Sweets
USE SPARINGLY

Milk, Yogurt
& Cheese Group
2-3 SERVINGS

Meat, Poultry, Fish
Dry Beans, Eggs
& Nuts Group
2-3 SERVINGS

Vegetable Group
3-5 SERVINGS

Fruit Group
2-4 SERVINGS

Bread, Cereal
Rice & Pasta Group
6-11 SERVINGS

The Spinning 8-Week Weight Loss Program is not about counting calories. However, it is helpful to have knowledge of the different food groups, what is considered a serving size, the macronutrients (carbohydrate, fat and protein) and calorie content. The easiest, quickest way is to learn how the food guide pyramid created by the United States Department of Agriculture (USDA) was used to develop diabetic exchange lists. The goal of diabetic exchange lists is to group foods by carbohydrate, protein, fat and calorie content in order to help individuals with diabetes choose foods that will allow them to control their blood sugar levels. After reviewing these lists, you will be more knowledgeable about the nutrition that specific foods contain. You will also gain a better understanding of what is considered a portion, which is a crucial component of weight loss success.

Grains and Starchy Vegetables Group
(Bread, Cereal, Rice and Pasta)

80 calories per serving: 15 grams of carbohydrate, 3 grams of protein, 0-1 gram of fat

One serving is equal to: 1/2 cup of pasta, 1/3 cup of rice, 3/4 to 1 ounce of cereal, 1 slice of bread, 1/2 of a small bagel, about 1/2 cup of starchy vegetables (potatoes, peas, corn)

Grain Tips: Choose grain products that list "whole" grain flour in the ingredient list. For example, if under the list of ingredients you see "wheat flour," the flour has been processed and the fiber and many of the nutrients have been taken out. If the term "whole wheat flour" is used, then the grain has been kept intact and there will be more fiber and nutrients per serving. Fiber is helpful for weight loss because it is filling and can decrease the number of calories the body absorbs. Also, try to choose grain products that have no added sugars. Ingredients such as sugar, liquid sugar, honey, sucrose, glucose, fructose and/or high fructose corn syrup indicate that sugar has been added. Many of these foods are listed as having more than 80 calories per serving, so you may need to adjust the serving size to the guidelines listed above. You may also note that 1/2 cup of pasta is one serving. That does not mean you can only have 1/2 a cup of pasta at a time. It just means that if you are going to eat 2 cups of pasta you need to realize that you are actually consuming four grain servings. You do not need to restrict your intake of starchy vegetables. They are natural—not processed—and are an excellent source of complex carbohydrates, fiber and phytonutrients.

Vegetable Group (excluding starchy vegetables)

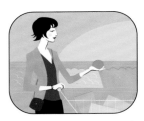

25 calories per serving: 5 grams of carbohydrate, 2 grams of protein, 0 grams of fat
One serving is equal to: 1/2 cup of cooked vegetables, 1 cup of raw vegetables
Vegetable Tips: Both raw and cooked vegetables are nutritious choices. Choose fresh or frozen instead of canned because canned vegetables have extra sodium added. Microwaving and steaming are the best cooking methods.

Fruit Group

60 calories per serving: 15 grams of carbohydrate, 0 grams of protein, 0 grams of fat
Serving sizes vary greatly—some examples include: 1/2 cup of orange juice, 1/2 banana, 1 orange, 1 apple, 1 1/4 cup of strawberries, 1/4 of a cantaloupe, 15 small grapes, 2 medium plums, 1 1/4 cup of watermelon, 1/2 of a grapefruit, 2 tablespoons of raisins.
Fruit Tips: It is better to get your fruit by eating pieces of fruit rather than relying on juice. Many people over-consume beverages. Juice is healthy, but drinking too much of it can hinder weight loss progress. Fruit takes longer to eat, contains fiber and is generally more nutritious and filling.

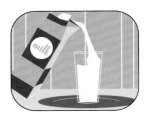

Dairy Group

A serving of skim milk contains: 90 calories, 12 grams of carbohydrate, 8 grams of protein, 1/2 gram of fat per serving
A serving of 1% fat milk contains: 100 calories, 12 grams of carbohydrate, 8 grams of protein, 2 grams of fat per serving
A serving of 2% fat milk contains: 120 calories, 12 grams of carbohydrate, 8 grams of protein, 5 grams of fat per serving
A serving of whole milk contains: 150 calories, 12 grams of carbohydrate, 8 grams of protein, 8 grams of fat per serving
One serving is equal to: 1 cup of milk, 1 cup of yogurt
Dairy Tips: Choose skim and low fat dairy products when possible.

Count fruit yogurt as 1 fruit and 1 dairy serving. Choose yogurts that have less added sugar. Avoid artificially sweetened yogurts and fat-free cheeses. According to diabetic exchange lists, cheese is considered a "meat" serving because of its protein and fat content.

Meat, Poultry, Dry Beans, Fish, Eggs and Nuts Group

One ounce of a lean meat contains: 55 calories, 0 grams of carbohydrate, 7 grams of protein, 3 grams of fat

One ounce of a medium-fat meat contains: 75 calories, 0 grams of carbohydrate, 7 grams of protein, 5 grams of fat

One ounce of a high-fat meat contains: 100 calories, 0 grams of carbohydrate, 7 grams of protein, 8 grams of fat

Lean meats include: chuck steak, flank steak, London broil, sandwich steaks, ham, Canadian bacon, chicken and turkey without skin, egg whites, drained can tuna, mackerel, crab, lobster, low-fat cottage cheese

Medium-fat meats include: ground beef (15% fat), roasts, steaks, rib eye steak, pork tenderloin, lamb, veal cutlet, chicken, duck and goose with skin, tuna, salmon, mozzarella cheese, ricotta cheese, soybeans, tofu, eggs

High-fat meats include: beef brisket, ground beef (>20% fat), Porterhouse steak, New York strip steak, most prime beefs, ground lamb, spare ribs, sausage, cheddar cheese, Roquefort, Swiss, gorgonzola, American cheese, peanut butter (add 1/2 bread exchange and 2 fat exchanges), peanuts, pumpkin seeds, cold cuts, pine nuts, hot dogs

Meat, Poultry, Dry Beans, Fish, Eggs and Nuts Tips: Choose lean meats whenever possible. People usually need less protein than they think. A healthy serving size is considered to be about 2-3 ounces of meat, poultry or fish; 1/2 cup of beans; 1 tablespoon of peanut butter; or approximately 4 tablespoons of seeds.

Fat Group

Many people equate losing weight with reducing or eliminating fat. Including fat in the diet provides several benefits:

• Increased feeling of fullness.
• Greater variety of food choices.
• Combined with Endurance and Recovery Energy Zone™ workouts, it can improve your body's ability to burn fat.
• Many foods that contain fat also contain protein and additional vitamins and minerals such as zinc, iron and vitamin B12 (which are all essential for optimal athletic performance).

You will experience better success if you choose fat-containing foods that also have additional nutrients. For example, natural peanut butter is a better choice than butter because butter is just pure fat and calories, while the natural peanut butter contains healthier types of fats and also provides protein and iron. The lists below will help you to decipher which types of foods contain healthier fats. (Remember that ALL fats contain 9 calories per gram.)

One serving contains: 45 calories, 0 grams of carbohydrate, 0 grams of protein, 5 grams of fat

One serving is equal to: 1 pat of butter, 1 teaspoon of any kind of oil, 1 tablespoon of most nuts, 1 tablespoon of cream cheese, 1 tablespoon of salad dressing, 2 teaspoons of mayonnaise

Fat tips: Olive oil, peanut oil and canola are the healthiest. Nuts and seeds are a good fat source, as well. The fats found in fatty fish such as tuna, salmon and mackerel are also considered healthy. Vegetable oil fats are second best. Animal fats, coconut oil and palm kernel oil are not as healthy. Hydrogenated and partially hydrogenated oils found in products like margarine and many processed foods are the absolute worst. Hydrogenated fats go through a process that makes them more solid and extends the shelf life of the products they are in. As a result of the hydrogenation process, they have been found to have the most negative effects on cholesterol levels and overall health. They cannot be processed by the body as easily as naturally occurring fats and are said to make fat and weight loss more difficult. Fully hydrogenated fats are as unhealthful as partially hydrogenated fats. When you shop, read the ingredient label.

> Be aware that many frozen, breaded foods and french fries have been pre-fried before they were frozen.

If you see the terms hydrogenated fat, trans-fatty acids, partially hydrogenated fat or shortening, try to find an alternative product without those ingredients listed. Avoid deep-fried foods as much as possible. Be aware that many frozen, breaded foods and french fries have been pre-fried before they were frozen. Virtually all of them contain hydrogenated fats. Minimizing your consumption of hydrogenated fats will lead you to choose more natural, less processed, lower calorie, more healthy foods. Most importantly, limiting all types of hydrogenated fats will improve your health and facilitate weight loss.

Choosing Healthy Foods

It's easy to know that you need to eat healthy foods, but it's not always easy to identify which foods are healthy. Choosing healthy foods is an important part of achieving weight loss success. Many food products that advertise the words "diet" or "low fat" are full of industrialized fats that can harm your body and hamper your weight loss progress. This section will teach you the difference between whole foods and real foods, processed foods and unprocessed foods, and hydrogenated fat and trans fat.

Real and Whole Foods

Real food is simply food that has been around for thousands of years, and has been prepared by traditional methods that have also existed for many years. The way the food is farmed, processed, prepared and cooked needs to be taken into consideration when you're looking to eat real foods.

As Michael Pollan, author of *In Defense Of* states, "If it wasn't around when your great grandparents were alive, don't eat it." And considering all of the new health complications of today, there seems to be quite a bit of validity to that statement.

Whole foods are foods that are not processed or refined in any way, and do not have any added ingredients. Some examples of whole foods include fresh produce, dairy, whole grains, meat and fish. Therefore, food that appears in its most pure form with minimal processing can be considered a whole food.

Processed vs. Unprocessed Foods

According to the Farm Bill of 2008, a processed food is one that has been processed to the point that it undergoes a "change of character." Examples of unprocessed vs. processed foods include:

- Raw nuts (unprocessed) vs. roasted nuts (processed)
- Edamame (unprocessed) vs. tofu (processed)
- Head of spinach (unprocessed) vs. cut, pre-washed spinach (processed)

While there is nothing wrong with roasting some nuts, creating tofu out of soybeans or cutting up and washing a head of spinach; this standard processing of ingredients involves scientifically altering the chemical structure of those foods. And it is unlikely that the chemical structure of a natural food could be changed without having some type of unexpected health consequence on us and our bodies.

Below are a couple of examples of scientifically altered (or processed) foods:

Recipe for margarine (from "Real Food" by Nina Planck):

• Begin with a polyunsaturated, liquid vegetable oil rancid from extraction under high heat. Mix with tiny metal particles, usually nickel oxide. In a high-pressure, high-temperature reactor, shoot hydrogen atoms at the unsaturated carbon bonds. Add soap-like emulsifiers and starch to make it soft and creamy. Steam to remove foul odors, bleach away the gray color, dye it yellow and add artificial flavors.

If you like butter, but want a healthier version, try mixing 1 stick of butter and 1/2 cup of extra virgin olive oil or 1/2 cup of organic canola oil in a blender, mix, and store in the refrigerator. The result is a spread that has the taste of real butter, with a higher monounsaturated (healthy) fat content that is more spreadable, making it easier to use less of it.

Recipe for typical commercial salt (from "Real Food" by Nina Planck):

• First, the chemical industry removes the valuable trace elements and heats it to 1200 degrees Fahrenheit. What's left is 100% sodium chloride, plus industrial additives, including aluminum, anti-caking agents, and dextrose, which stains it purple. Salt is then bleached. Consuming pure sodium chloride strains the body, upsetting fluid balance and dehydrating cells.

Recipe for white flour:

Whole grains are made up of three components:

• Bran, which is the protective coat which contains fiber and minerals.
• Endosperm, which is carbohydrate wrapped in protein.
• Germ, which is the tiny seed that contains fat, protein and vitamins.

During processing, the bran and germ are stripped from the grain, leaving the endosperm (which contains mostly carbohydrates and some B vitamins). The most nutrition is in the germ and bran. Many companies enrich the processed flour in an attempt to restore some of the nutrition that has been lost, but never to the level of the original grain. What is left behind is a carbohydrate-containing product that is digested similarly to a simple sugar, which provides low nutrition and short-term satiety.

The motivation for processing and creating preservatives with fat and sugar substitutes stems from a combination of an unwillingness by consumers to spend time on food preparation and the desire for them to achieve results (whether it be weight loss or better health) without having to give up their reliance on consuming products.

Achieving long term weight loss and better health involves spending time preparing food, and the willingness to reduce your intake of sugars and unhealthy fats by choosing healthy, real foods, instead. There are no short cuts.

Hydrogenated Fats vs. Trans Fats

Great strides were made in the food labeling industry in January of 2006. Companies were suddenly required to disclose the amount of trans fat that was contained in their products, under the 'Nutrition Facts' section of the standard food label.

For many years, food processing plants had been using something called hydrogenated fats in the making of food products. To achieve this, chemists would start with a vegetable oil or soybean oil (which has a large number of double-bonds between the carbon atoms and are also known as polyunsaturated fats). They then discovered that if they added hydrogen atoms to the unsaturated carbon atoms, the consistency of the oil would become more solid and the shelf life of the food would be extended. When normal fat goes through this hydrogenation process, its atoms are rearranged, thus turning it into trans fat.

Consuming trans fats causes unexpected health problems including (but not limited to) weight gain (beyond calorie balance), weight gain around the waist, increased blood pressure, unfavorable cholesterol levels, elevated blood-sugar levels and higher blood pressure.

So, in an attempt to educate consumers, the term "trans fat" has been added to nutrition labels. And since 2006, companies are required to inform consumers about how many grams of trans fat each serving of their product contains.

However, that isn't the whole story. Some fats that undergo hydrogenation do not form any trans bonds, so they cannot be referred to as a "trans fats." Yet, they still went through a chemical process which resulted in a change in their structure. To further complicate matters, there are naturally occurring trans fats in some beef and dairy products. These naturally occurring fats are unfairly grouped with artificially produced trans fats, under current standard labeling policies.

Companies can produce products that contain up to a half-of-a-gram of fat and up to half-of-a-gram of trans fat per serving, and they can still advertise their product as being "trans-fat free."

Our goal intake of hydrogenated fats per day is of course 0 grams, but if you insist on eating hydrogenated fat-containing foods, the suggested limit is 2 grams per day. And even if you consume many trans-fat free products (each containing up to a half-of-a-gram per serving) that could still easily add up to a dangerously high amount of trans fats in your diet.

Before reviewing hydrogenated fat identification information, you need to know about a new, dangerous type of fat called "interesterified fat." An inter-esterified fat is one that started out as a polyunsaturated fat and went through the full process of hydrogenation. Remember, fats that are fully hydrogenated are very solid. This makes them difficult to work with when try-ing to create appealing food products. Therefore, chemists have learned that if they put fully hydrogenated fats through a few more processes, they will become less solid and more product-friendly. This means that over-processed trans fat (that is made to be soft), is "interesterified fat."

You can find interesterified fats on the ingredient lists of products like wraps and burrito shells. Companies have started using them more often because they do not contribute to a foods "trans fat" content, and they still extend product shelf life (because they are derived from trans fats). Since they have gone through the hydrogenation process, they may also contribute to health problems like increased blood sugar levels.

Below are examples of a few standard food labels. You can see that the product on the left contains 0 trans fats and that there are no hydrogenated fats listed on its ingredient list. The product on the right contains 3 grams of trans fats and partially hydrogenated fat is third on the ingredient list.

Obviously, the product on the left is the healthier choice of the two.

Nutrition Facts		
Serving Size 2 oz. (56g/ 1 bar)		
Servings per container 1		
Amount Per Serving		
Calories 150 Calories from Fat 90		
	% Daily Value	
Total Fat 10g	**15%**	
Saturated Fat 6g	**30%**	
Trans Fat 0g		
Ingredients: Whole oats, sugar, butter, salt.		

Nutrition Facts		
Serving Size 2 oz. (56g/ 1 bar)		
Servings per container 1		
Amount Per Serving		
Calories 150 Calories from Fat 90		
	% Daily Value	
Total Fat 10g	**15%**	
Saturated Fat 3g	**15%**	
Trans Fat 3g		
Ingredients: Oatmeal, sugar, partially hydrogenat-ed soybean oil, sugar, food starch, salt.		

You may find that some products that contain "0 grams of trans fat" still have hydrogenated, partially hydrogenated or interesterified fats on their ingredient lists.

To avoid consumption of the unhealthiest industrialized fats, you must ignore trans-fat free claims on the front of the package (and the fact that the product may have the number zero listed next to the amount of trans fat). Instead, scan ingredient lists on everything that you consume. If you see the words hydrogenated, partially hydrogenated or interesterified, then find something else to buy.

Striving to eliminate hydrogenated fats from your diet will motivate you to prepare more of your own foods and enable you to identify some of the healthier convenience foods. Equally as important, you will be sending the message to food manufacturers that food quality matters to you.

Changing Your Diet: An Example

A 50 year-old, 5'4" woman weighed 160 pounds and struggled with weight loss, even after working with a personal trainer for a full year, lifting weights 3 times a week, attending Spinning® classes, and cycling outdoors (sometimes for as long as 30 miles). Although she improved her body composition, she was frustrated that her weight was stuck at 160 pounds.

After keeping a record of everything she ate for one week, diet analysis revealed that she consumed an average of approximately 1,200 calories per day, and her diet was low in protein, fiber, Vitamin A, Vitamin E, calcium and potassium.

Below is a sample of what her typical diet looked like:

Breakfast: 1 diet bar, 1 cup of yogurt, 1 cup of sugar-free French vanilla coffee

Lunch: 1 microwavable southwest-style chicken panini, 1 cup of cranberry juice

Dinner: Large salad with iceberg lettuce, feta cheese, grape tomatoes, cucumbers with fat-free Caesar dressing

Snacks: Peanut butter, peaches with fat-free whipped cream, 1 diet bar, 1 fat-free pudding cup

She hardly ever cooked and almost everything she consumed was a "diet" or "light" convenience food. These products featured extensive ingredient lists (many of which were unrecognizable). The beverages she consumed were primarily coffee with diet creamer and diet juices. With her calorie intake being so low already, it was not best to further restrict her caloric intake. Instead, it was encouraged that she increase the amount of fiber in her diet, eat more whole foods and consume fewer diet foods.

Below is a list of her main dietary goals:

• Drink at least 40 ounces of water/day. The typical recommendation is 64 ounces, but since she was hardly drinking any, she wanted to start with a goal that was more achievable.
• Snack on raw carrots (or other vegetables) instead of diet bars. Ironically, she used to snack on carrots, but after reading in a popular diet book that carrots contained a lot of sugar, she replaced them with diet bars from the same branded diet program. At 100 calories each, consuming 3-4 per day, she could be eating an extra meal with real food for the same caloric content, each day.
• Avoid snacking after dinner. This goal was especially important since most of the foods she ate after dinner were treats, low in nutrition and high in hydrogenated fats.
• Add one calcium serving daily. Improving one's diet is not just about calorie reduction/weight loss, but also about improving nutrition content. Finding a balance between reducing unhealthy foods and increasing intake of better quality foods will further contribute to long term success.

The woman worked hard at these goals for 5 weeks, and committed to eating whole foods rather than "diet" foods. After completing a new week's worth of food records, these were the results:

Breakfast: Fat-free organic plain yogurt with raspberries, whole oat toast with natural peanut butter, 1 cup of French vanilla coffee

Lunch: Whole wheat wrap with chicken, part-skim cheese, lettuce, peppers, tomatoes, 1% milk

Dinner: Large salad with romaine lettuce, feta cheese, grape tomatoes, orange peppers, cucumbers with olive oil and balsamic vinegar

Snacks: peaches with fat-free whipped cream, 1 diet bar, baby carrots with hummus, 47 ounces of water

There were a couple of unhealthy foods (coffee and whipped cream) that she refused to give up at that time, but aside from that, she made many significant improvements. She routinely increased her water intake to 50 ounces per day, decreased her diet bar intake to one per day, snacked on baby carrots and other raw vegetables and replaced frozen dinners with simple, fresh meals that she prepared herself.

Upon further analysis, it was determined that the only nutrients that her diet was low in were Vitamin E, calcium and potassium (although levels of these nutrients had increased when compared to the first diet analysis). Her exercise routine remained consistent, and her average caloric intake increased to 1,300 a day, but as a result of her revised diet, she lost 8 pounds in 5 weeks.

Let's take a closer look at the ingredients that are in the natural foods she ate versus the ingredients that are in the diet foods that she ate:

Diet Food	Ingredient List	Natural Food	Ingredient List
Diet Bar	Multi-grain crisp (whole grain wheat flour, degermed yellow cornmeal, whole grain oat flour, salt), maltilol syrup, rolled oats, whole grain barley, whole grain wheat, oligofructose (for fiber), sugar, brown rice syrup, soy protein isolate, fractionated palm kernel oil, partially de-fatted peanut oil, evaporated cane juice, invert syrup, rice flour, inulin (for fiber), glycerin, cream, natural flavor (contains peanuts), non-fat milk, butter (cream, salt), salt, vegetable oil (palm kernel and palm oil), cocoa, milk pro tein isolate, sodium caseinate, soy lecithin, barley, malt, whey, sodium phosphate, carrageenan, erythritol, sucralose, artificial flavor, tocopherols and caramel color.	Carrots Hummus	Carrots Chickpeas, tahini, garlic, lemon juice, canola oil, salt
Sugar Free Low-Calorie Syrup	Water, sorbitol, natural & artificial maple flavor (sulfites), cellulose gum, sucralose, salt, potassium sorbate and sodium benzoate, citric acid, caramel color (sulfites), acesulfame, potassium, zinc, lactate, niacinamide, D-calcium pantothenate, pyridoxine, hydrochloride, thiamin, mononi trate, cyanocobalumin (gluten-free)	Pure Maple Syrup	100% Pure Maple Syrup
Cranberry Juice	Filtered water, cranberry juice from concentrate and cranberry juice, fructose, pectin, natural flavors, sodium citrate, acesul fame, potassium, sucralose	Orange Juice (not from concentrate)	Oranges from Florida and Brazil
Yogurt	Cultured, pasteurized grade A non-fat milk, blueberries, fructose, modified food starch, kosher gela tin, natural flavors, malic acid, aspartame, potassium sorbate, red 40, blue 1, live active yogurt cultures including bifidus BB-12	Low-Fat Vanilla Yogurt	Cultured pasteurized organic low fat milk, naturally milled organic sugar, organic natural vanilla flavor, pectin, vitamin D3, contains our exclusive blend of six live active yogurt cultures including l. aciophilus, bifidus, l. casei AND l. rhamnosus.

Diet Food	Ingredient List	Natural Food	Ingredient List
Frozen Dinner	Cooked white meat chicken (white meat chicken, water, modified tapioca starch, sugar, salt, sodium phosphate, glazed with water, caramel coloring, modified potato starch), yellow zucchini, zucchini, water, red bell peppers, roasted garlic puree, (garlic, high maltose corn syrup solids), contains 2% or less of: chicken fat, margarine (soybean oil, water, salt, partially hydrogenated soy bean oil, mono- and diglycerides, soy lecithin, sodium benzoate, natural flavor, artificial flavor, beta carotene (color), vitamin A palmitate), modified cornstarch, onions, spice, salt, garlic puree, chicken type flavor, (flavor, autolyzed yeast extract, chicken fat (bha, propyl concentrate, xanthan gum, chicken flavor, (autolyzed yeast extract, chicken broth, water, salt, flavor), black pepper, concentrated onion juice (onion juice, sunflower oil), sucralose, citric, sodium citrate).	White Chicken-Chili	Cannellini beans, chicken broth, garbanzo beans, chicken, yellow onion, chili powder, garlic, soy sauce

After reviewing the information from the table above, you can see that it is important to be aware of what foods you are putting into your body. To learn more about some of the additives in the foods listed above, you can read the newsletter article titled "Chemical Cuisine" at: *www.cspinet.org/nah/05_08/chem_cuisine.pdf.* The article lists food additives that are found in many packaged foods. These additives are categorized in the following groups:

• Safe
• Cut Back (not toxic, but large amounts may be unsafe or unhealthy)
• Caution (may pose a risk and needs to be better tested)
• Certain people should avoid
• Everyone Should Avoid (unsafe or very poorly tested and not worth any risk)

The number of ingredients that fall into the latter three categories and are abundantly used in packaged foods is astounding. And in some cases, they are even more prevalent in foods that are marketed as being "healthy."

It would be fair to expect that if an ingredient is in the "Everyone Should Avoid" category, then no one in the food industry should be able to produce it. But you will be surprised to find that all artificial sweeteners (with the exception of sucralose) are in the "Everyone Should Avoid" category (and even sucralose needs further testing before a final verdict can be determined). You will find that hydrogenated fats (the fats that you earn big points for avoiding in this program) also fall into the "Everyone Should Avoid" category.

It has been said that people today no longer eat food, we eat products. Your best approach to better health involves eating more real foods and whole foods, and fewer 'products.'

Menu Makeovers

There are many ways you can improve your diet. One way is to eat healthier alternatives of your regular favorites. The following Menu Makeovers provide examples of foods that you might eat throughout the day, and how they can be changed into healthier substitutes that you can feel good about.

You might find that some or many of the items listed under the "Before" columns of these menus are currently a part of your daily diet. If so, consider making the recommended substitutions. Remember, healthier eating is a key factor in acheiving maintainable weight loss success.

Once you have reviewed the Menu Makeover examples, see if you can make similar substitutes in your daily diet. Or, simply browse the items listed in the "After" columns of the menus to find good ideas for healthy snacks and meals that you can prepare for yourself.

Makeover #1

MENU	BEFORE	AFTER
Breakfast	• Sweetened "O's" cereal • Whole milk • Coffee with non-dairy creamer and sugar	• Unsweetened "O's" cereal • 1% Milk • 1 Pear • Water (12 oz.) • Coffee with cinnamon and 1% milk
Snack	Cereal bar	• 1 Banana • (16 oz.)
Lunch	• Turkey, ham and cheese on white bread with mayonnaise • Soda • 100-calorie snack packs	• Turkey breast with a slice of part-skim cheese on whole grain bread with lettuce, tomato, red onion and Dijon mustard • Side salad with balsamic vinegar and a small amount of extra virgin olive oil • Seltzer water (12 oz.)
Snack	Bag of pretzels	• 1 Small whole wheat pita pocket cut into triangles and toasted • Seltzer water (12 oz.)
Dinner	• Hamburger • French fries • Milkshake	• Ground sirloin (grass-fed) on a whole grain roll with lettuce, tomato and red onion • Steamed broccoli (1 cup) • Homemade shake with plain or vanilla yogurt, milk and strawberries

Makeover #2

MENU	BEFORE	AFTER
Breakfast	• Instant oatmeal (maple and brown sugar flavored) • Whole milk • Coffee with non-dairy creamer and artificial sweetener	• Steel cut oats with flaxseeds, raisins and cinnamon • 1% Milk • Water (16 oz.)
Snack	• Peanut butter crackers (packaged)	• Banana with natural peanut butter • Water (16 oz.)
Lunch	• Broccoli Cheese Soup • Yogurt • Fruit pack • Diet soda	• Butternut squash soup • Cashews • 1 cup of plain yogurt with vanilla extract (added for flavor) and frozen blueberries • Water (16 oz.)
Snack	• Diet energy bar • Iced tea (sugar added)	• Vegan, gluten and dairy-free snack bar • Seltzer water (8 oz.)
Dinner	• Baked breaded chicken • Peas • White rice • Flavored water (containing artificial sweetener)	• Roasted chicken with roasted root vegetables (onions, carrots, potatoes, and celery) • Brown rice • Seltzer water (8 oz.)

Makeover #3

MENU	BEFORE	AFTER
Breakfast	• Scrambled eggs (cooked in margarine) • Sausage • Coffee with artificial sweetener and non-dairy creamer	• 2 egg omelet with part-skim mozzarella cheese, spinach, onions and mushrooms • 1% Milk • 1 Peach • Water (16 oz.)
Snack	• Saltines • Soda	• Whole grain crackers • 8 ounces of seltzer water • 1 mug of herbal tea
Lunch	• Beef & bean chili • Macaroni • Sweetened applesauce • Diet iced tea	• Vegetarian chili (with beans, tomato, onions, & corn) • 1 apple • Water (16 oz.)
Snack	• Nachos with melted cheese and salsa	• Raw red & green pepper strips and salsa • 8 ounces of water
Dinner	• 7-layer burrito with beans, ground beef, cheese, guacamole, salsa, cheese and sour cream • Soda	• Black bean burritos on whole wheat burrito shells with part-skim cheese, spinach, garlic, onion, carrots, sweet potato and peppers • Brown rice & salsa • 16 ounces of seltzer water

Makeover #4

MENU	BEFORE	AFTER
Breakfast	• Raspberry yogurt • White toast with jelly • Sweetened juice	• Plain yogurt (flavored with vanilla extract) and frozen raspberries • Whole grain toast with apple butter (no sugar added) • Water (16 oz.)
Snack	• Small package of chips • Diet soda	• Raw almonds (1 oz) • 8 ounces of water
Lunch	• Hot dog • Baked beans • Canned fruit (in heavy syrup) • Sweetened iced tea	• Salad with sunflower seeds, cucumbers, shredded carrots, raisins • Whole grain roll • 1 cup of mixed fruit • Water (16 oz.)
Snack	• Baked potato chips	• Trail mix (made with plain nuts and fruit; no sugar or preservatives added) • Water (16 oz.)
Dinner	• White pasta with marinara sauce • Side salad with creamy Italian dressing • 20 ounce fruit drink	• Homemade pesto on whole grain pasta. • Small side salad with white balsamic vinegar and a little bit of extra virgin olive oil • Water (16 oz.)

Makeover #5

MENU	BEFORE	AFTER
Breakfast	• Sugary cereal (with dehydrated, sweetened strawberries) • Whole milk • Large glass of juice	• Shredded wheat cereal • Ground flaxseeds • 1% Milk • 1 cup of fresh mixed berries • Water (16 oz.)
Snack	• Packaged, pre-popped popcorn • 12 ounces of diet soda	• Air-popped popcorn • Water (8 oz.)
Lunch	• Chicken nuggets • Fries • Orange fruit drink	• Stir-fry chicken, carrots, onions and peppers • Brown rice • Orange • Water (8 oz.)
Snack	• Gummy bears	• Cherry tomatoes • Water (8 oz.)
Dinner	• Meatballs with marinara sauce over white pasta • Small salad with iceberg lettuce and creamy Ranch dressing • Diet iced tea	• Steak kabobs - sirloin steak, mushrooms, peppers, onions, cherry tomatoes • Brown rice • Small salad with homemade dressing (balsamic vinegar, extra virgin olive oil, garlic, chopped fresh basil) • 16 ounces of seltzer

Makeover #6

MENU	BEFORE	AFTER
Breakfast	• Cream of wheat (with sugar added) • Whole milk • Large glass of juice	• Whole grain cream of wheat • 1% milk • Mixed fresh berries • Water (16 oz.)
Snack	• Energy bar	• Vegan, gluten and dairy-free snack bar • Water (8 oz.)
Lunch	• Hamburger on white roll with ketchup and mayonnaise • French fries • Soda	• Black bean burger (vegetarian) on a whole grain roll • Salsa • Mixed fruit salad and cottage cheese
Snack	• White bread with peanut butter (containing hydrogenated fat)	• Sliced apples and natural almond butter • Seltzer water (8 oz.)
Dinner	• Breaded and fried fish • Green beans (with margarine added) • Baked (white) potato • Fruit drink	• Broiled salmon • Broiled or grilled asparagus in garlic and a small amount of extra virgin olive oil • Roasted sweet potatoes • Water (16 oz.)

Makeover #7

MENU	BEFORE	AFTER
Breakfast	• Box mix pancakes with maple syrup • Sausage links • Orange slices • 8 ounces of whole milk • Coffee with non-dairy creamer and sugar	• Homemade pancakes (made with whole grain flour) and topped with mashed bananas • Applesauce topped with yogurt and cinnamon • Sliced mangos • 1% milk (8 oz)
Snack	• Mixed, salted nuts • Diet iced tea	• Walnuts (1/2 cup) • Raisins (1 cup) • Water (8 oz.)
Lunch	• Grilled cheese sandwich on white bread (cooked in margarine) • 1 tomato slice • Canned tomato soup • Fruit drink	• Whole grain pita pocket stuffed with hummus, shredded carrots, red onion, shredded lettuce • Vegetarian vegetable soup (homemade) • Water (16 oz.)
Snack	• Canned fruit in heavy syrup	• Mixed fruit with low fat cottage cheese • Water (8 oz.)
Dinner	• Battered and fried shrimp over linguini (made with white/processed flour) • Caesar salad with croutons • Iced tea with lemon and sugar	• Scallops with stewed tomatoes, white wine, garlic and broccoli served over whole grain angel hair pasta • Side salad with homemade dressing • Water (16 oz.)

Makeover #8

MENU	BEFORE	AFTER
Breakfast	• Frozen blueberry waffles with maple syrup and margarine • Juice from concentrate	• Homemade whole grain waffles topped with sliced strawberries and yogurt • 1/2 grapefruit • Water (16 oz.)
Snack	• Chewy granola bar dipped in chocolate	• Trail mix (plain nuts and dried fruit: no added sugar or preservatives) • Water (8 oz.)
Lunch	• Diet frozen fish dinner • Side salad with Thousand Island dressing • Fruit drink	• Grilled shrimp sautéed in garlic and olive oil • Steamed green beans • Brown rice • Fruit cup • Seltzer water (16 oz.)
Snack	• Chips dipped in Ranch dressing • Water flavored with an artificial sweetener	• Raw sugar snap peas • Hummus • Water (8 oz.)
Dinner	• Turkey burger on a white roll • Sweet potato fries • 1 Tomato slice • Soda	• Autumn vegetable stew with butternut squash, chickpeas, stewed tomatoes, sweet potatoes, onion, garlic, turmeric • Couscous • Water (16 oz.)

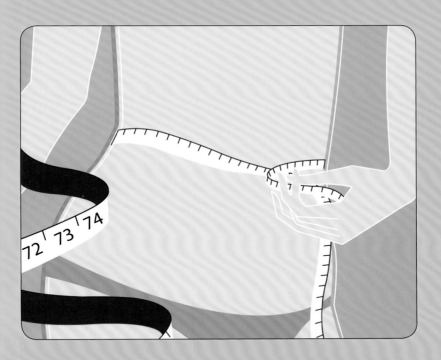

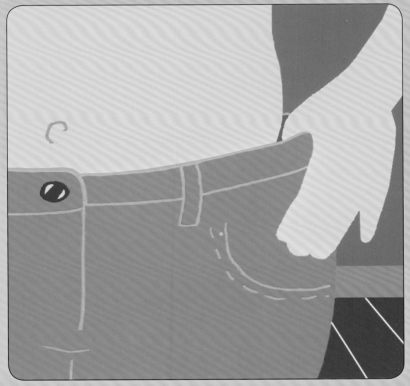

Heart Rate Training

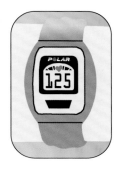

Now that you've learned some important fundamentals about nutrition, let's focus on the other component of your Spinning® 8-Week Weight Loss Program: exercise. The most fundamental message is simply to make exercise part of your routine. But beyond that, there's something very important to learn: heart rate training. It may sound advanced or complicated, but it's really quite simple. When we talk about heart rate training, we're talking about exercising at the right intensity for burning fat, strengthening your cardiovascular system, or whatever your exercise goals are. And your heart rate is the indicator that will tell you when you're exercising at the right intensity.

Heart Rate Monitors

There are a couple of tools you can use to let you know what your heart rate is during exercise: heart rate monitors and rating of perceived exertion. In the past you may have simply counted your pulse, but that method isn't accurate enough. Counting your pulse requires you to slow down your exercise activity, which causes your heart rate to immediately drop. Using the method of perceived exertion is very simple, but not always specific enough on its own. You can get the best feedback regarding training intensity by combining the perceived exertion method with the use of a heart rate monitor.

Perceived Exertion Chart

	Description	Energy Zone™	Heart Rate
Easy	Very little or light effort. You could maintain this pace for a long time.	Recovery	50-65%
Moderate	A moderate, completely aerobic pace. It's a pace that does not leave you breathless; you can still talk while at this exertion level.	Endurance	65-75%
Hard	Comfortably hard (athletes would call it threshold). Breathing is harder, so talking is possible, but you have to pause for breaths between phrases.	Strength	75-86%
Very Hard	This is the highest exertion level that you could reach. You could maintain this pace only for a short time. Talking would be very uncomfortable and difficult.	Race Day	85-92%

Heart Rate Training Zones

Before you can use heart rate training, you'll need to know what your target heart rate zones (ranges) are. You have seen heart rate charts up on the wall at your gym that indicate zones based on your age. There are several problems with those charts:

1. People of the same age do not necessarily have the same target heart rates.

2. The charts do not take current level of fitness or any other health considerations into account.

3. They assume that all younger people have higher target heart rates than older people (and vice versa).

4. They do not take the resting heart rate into account, which can result in heart rate ranges that are too low and/or too broad.

Another method of determining target heart rates consists of trying to find your true maximum heart rate by either noting what your highest heart rate was during a very hard workout or doing a maximum heart rate test. There are a few problems with this as well:

1. It is inappropriate and unsafe for many people to try to push themselves up to their maximum heart rate.

2. Maximum heart rate tests are usually too short to get an accurate maximum heart rate test result.

3. In many cases, an individual's maximum heart rate may be about 10 beats or so higher than what they see during their hardest workout.

For these reasons, in this program, we'll use a heart rate chart that determines your heart rate training zones based on your resting heart rate and anaerobic threshold heart rate.

1. **Determine your resting heart rate** by taking your pulse just before you fall asleep or before you get out of bed in the morning. You can either strap on a heart rate monitor or find your pulse in your wrist and count for a full minute. Do this about 3-5 consecutive mornings and calculate the average. This will give you an accurate resting heart rate.

2. **Determine your anaerobic threshold.** Your anaerobic threshold is the point at which you are exercising so hard that your body has to rely on producing some of its energy without oxygen. When your body has to produce energy anaerobically, by-products such as carbon dioxide and

lactic acid build up to the point that you will start to feel fatigue in the muscles and you will notice your breathing rate increase. If you continue to exercise beyond this point, you will feel distinctly uncomfortable. If you are doing this program with a group, your Program Leader will lead you through an anaerobic threshold test at the beginning of the program. If you are doing this program on your own, you can make an appointment with a certified fitness professional who is qualified to administer the AT test for you.

3. Once you know these two key numbers, you can use the following charts to find out what your target heart rate ranges are. When you refer to the charts, choose the one with the resting heart rate that is closest to yours. Then select the row with the heart rate in bold that is closest to your anaerobic threshold.

Example: If your resting heart rate is 62 and your anaerobic threshold is 170, you will find your target heart rate ranges in the second table, sixth row:

Recovery Energy Zone™	Endurance Energy Zone	Strength Energy Zone	Interval	Interval Recovery	Race Day Energy Zone
125-145	145-158	158-171	171-180	138	164-180

How to interpret these numbers: With the above example, for the Endurance Energy Zone, your heart rate should stay between 145 and 158 beats per minute (BPM). Your heart rate monitor will continuously display your heart rate, making it easy for you to know if you're exercising too hard or too light.

Spinning® Energy Zone™ Charts

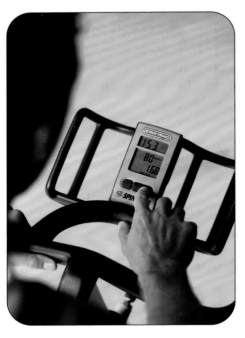

The following three charts provide heart rate zones based on your AT heart rate and resting heart rate. If you do not know those numbers you may also use the age-based heart rate chart that follows.

First select the chart with the resting heart rate closest to your own. Then select the row with the AT heart rate closest to your own. That row will give you your heart rate ranges for each Energy Zone. Note: The AT heart rate matches the upper end of the Strength Energy Zone. Record your heart rate zones in your log book for easy reference. You will need to refer to these numbers each time you take part in a Spinning® ride.

RESTING HEART RATE: 50						
Lactate Threshold Heart Rate	Recovery Energy Zone	Endurance Energy Zone	Strength Energy Zone	Intense Interval	Interval Recovery	Race Day Energy Zone
148	108-125	125-136	136-148	148-156	119	142-156
152	110-128	128-140	140-152	152-160	122	146-160
156	113-131	131-144	144-156	156-165	125	150-165
161	115-135	135-148	148-161	161-170	128	154-170
165	118-138	138-151	151-165	165-174	131	158-174
169	120-141	141-155	155-169	169-179	134	162-179
173	123-144	144-159	159-173	173-183	137	166-183
178	125-148	148-163	163-178	178-188	140	170-188
182	128-151	151-166	166-182	182-193	143	174-193
186	130-154	154-170	170-186	186-197	146	178-197

RESTING HEART RATE: 60

Lactate Threshold Heart Rate	Recovery Energy Zone	Endurance Energy Zone	Strength Energy Zone	Intense Interval	Interval Recovery	Race Day Energy Zone
149	113-128	128-139	139-149	149-157	123	144-157
154	115-132	132-143	143-154	154-161	126	148-161
158	118-135	135-146	146-158	158-166	129	152-166
162	120-138	138-150	150-162	162-170	132	156-170
166	123-141	141-154	154-166	166-175	135	160-175
171	125-145	145-158	158-171	171-180	138	164-180
175	128-148	148-161	161-175	175-184	141	168-184
179	130-151	151-165	165-179	179-189	144	172-189
183	133-154	154-169	169-183	183-193	147	176-193
188	135-158	158-173	173-188	188-198	150	180-198

RESTING HEART RATE: 70

Lactate Threshold Heart Rate	Recovery Energy Zone	Endurance Energy Zone	Strength Energy Zone	Intense Interval	Interval Recovery	Race Day Energy Zone
151	118-132	132-141	141-151	151-157	127	146-157
155	120-135	135-145	145-155	155-162	130	150-162
159	123-138	138-149	149-159	159-167	133	154-167
164	125-142	142-153	153-164	164-171	136	158-171
168	128-145	145-156	156-168	168-176	139	162-176
172	130-148	148-160	160-172	172-180	142	166-180
176	133-151	151-164	164-176	176-185	145	170-185
181	135-155	155-168	168-181	181-190	148	174-190
185	138-158	158-171	171-185	185-194	151	178-194
189	140-161	161-175	175-189	189-199	154	182-199

ENERGY ZONE™ HEART RATE CHART

AGE	RECOVERY 50-65%	ENDURANCE 65-75%	STRENGTH 75-85%	INTERVAL 65-92%	RACE DAY 80-92%
20-23	100-129	129-149	149-168	129-182	160-182
24-27	98-126	126-146	146-165	126-178	155-178
28-31	96-123	123-143	143-162	123-175	153-175
32-35	94-120	120-140	140-159	120-172	150-172
36-39	92-118	118-137	137-155	118-168	146-168
40-43	90-116	116-134	134-151	116-164	143-164
44-47	88-113	113-131	131-148	113-161	140-162
48-51	86-110	110-128	128-145	110-157	137-157
52-55	84-108	108-125	125-141	108-153	133-153
56-60	82-105	105-122	122-139	105-150	131-150

Example: If you're 30 years old, your target heart rate for the Endurance Energy Zone is 123–143 beats per minute.

Energy Zone™ Benefits

There are specific fitness improvements that happen as a result of training in each specific Energy Zone:

1. Recovery Energy Zone
- 50-65% of maximum heart rate
- Used for warm-ups, cool-downs and rejuvenation of the body.
- Especially useful for less-conditioned individuals who are brand new to exercise, and for well-conditioned competitive athletes who like to train 6-7 days per week.

2. Endurance Energy Zone
- 65-75% of maximum heart rate
- Training in this zone results in increased aerobic capacity, fat-burning efficiency, and lung capacity; a stronger heart; fewer injuries; more energy; and a stronger immune system.
- Nearly everybody should spend more time training in the Endurance Energy Zone than in any other zone.

3. Strength Energy Zone
- 75-85% of maximum heart rate
- Training in this zone increases aerobic capacity, anaerobic capacity, anaerobic threshold (or the ability to do more work at the anaerobic threshold), ability to buffer lactic acid, and strength in tendons and ligaments.
- This zone is useful to those who have spent at least 8 weeks building an aerobic base.

4. Intense Interval and Race Day Energy Zones™
- Intense Interval = 85-92% of maximum heart rate with recovery heart rate at 60% of the maximum heart rate.
- Race Day = 80-92% of the maximum heart rate

Training in the Intense Interval/Race Day Energy Zones allows for the further development of speed, coordination, power and anaerobic fitness. Intense Interval and Race Day workouts are so intense that the metabolism typically stays elevated after the workout is over.

Intense Interval and Race Day rides are ideal for individuals who have spent plenty of time building an aerobic base, are comfortable working in the Strength Energy Zone, and are seeking significant improvements in performance. The term "interval" actually just refers to doing bouts of harder work interspersed with bouts of easier work. Even if you're not a competitive athlete, you can benefit dramatically from interval workouts after utilizing the Recovery, Endurance and Strength Energy Zones first.

Exercise Schedule

Now that you have completed your fitness tests and have learned about heart rate training, you have the knowledge you need to exercise in the zones appropriate for your fitness level. Your goal is to exercise 5 days per week, with three 40-minute Spinning rides. On the other two days, choose any exercise activity you want. Listed below are some activity intensity suggestions based on your current level of fitness.

1. Deconditioned: If you have not exercised in a long time or are very deconditioned, your goal is to just work on becoming active and keeping the exercise sessions comfortable. You should start by spending most of your training time in the Recovery Energy Zone™ and becoming consistent.

1. Somewhat New to Fitness: If you have been exercising, but not for very long, you should continue to work on building an aerobicic base. You should spend at least 80-90% of your total cardiovascular training time in the Endurance Energy Zone since that is where the greatest number of fitness benefits occur. Once you feel stronger, your workouts can be designed to include some time in the lower half of the Strength Energy Zone (75-80% of the maximum heart rate), which would still be considered working aerobically. Some Recovery Zone work can be beneficial, as well.

3. Developed a Good Aerobic Base: If you have already spent a minimum of 8 weeks developing your aerobic base, you are ready for the next level! Approximately 70% of your training time should be spent working in the Endurance Energy Zone, with 30% in the Strength Energy Zone. At this point, you can incorporate moderately intense interval workouts. However, it is suggested that you do your best to not go beyond 85% of your maximum heart rate during the interval workouts.

4. Seeking Enhanced Performance: If you have excellent fitness and you are ready to push your fitness to the next level, then this is the schedule for you:
Recovery Energy Zone = 5% of total training time
Endurance Energy Zone = 65% of total training time
Strength Energy Zone = 20% of total training time
Interval (you can incorporate more intense intervals into your schedule now) and Race Day Energy Zones = 10% of total training time.
Remember to include rest days and to give yourself adequate recovery time after more intense workouts.

Resistance training is a crucial component to better body composition. Weight lifting/resistance training 2-3 days a week is a good goal. If you have not lifted weights before, you should consider scheduling an appointment with a certified trainer who can help you develop a weight-lifting routine.

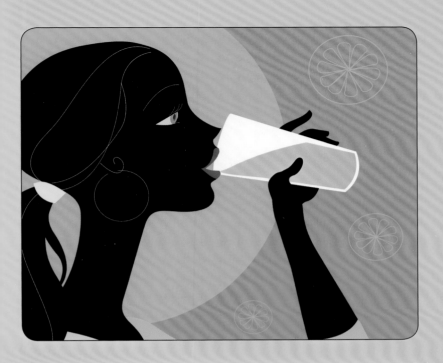
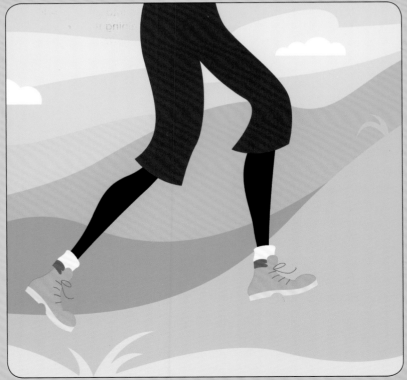

Healthy Habits Score Sheets

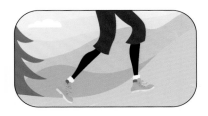

Now that you have a basic understanding of general nutrition and the principles of successful weight loss, you are ready to learn about the Healthy Habits tracking system. Together with your exercise routine, these habits are the keys to your fitness success. You have Healthy Habits score sheets for each week of the 8-week program. Each score sheet lists Healthy Habits that you should focus on for that day. You will begin the program with two Healthy Habits. Each week, two more Healthy Habits will be added until all eight habits are part of your daily lifestyle. This will happen by the end of Week Four. In the last four weeks, you will focus on as many of the eight habits simultaneously as you can.

At the beginning of each day, you will read the Healthy Habits so that you know what your nutrition goals are. Your goal is to follow the listed Habits and earn points. Habits with a greater number of points are generally more objective and may be more difficult to follow, but will make a greater impact on your weight loss, nutrition and health success. Complete the Healthy Habits score sheets that are located in your 8-Week Weight Loss Program Healthy Habits and Activity Score Sheets logbook every single day. The goal is to create a change in the way you eat. If you wait until the end of the week or the month and try to remember what you did, then you will not be guaranteed success.

> **Complete the Healthy Habits score sheets every day.**

It is okay if you are not able to follow every single habit every day. Do the best that you possibly can, and give yourself partial credit when you feel you deserve it. Remain positive, even when you don't earn perfect scores.

Cutting calories by making healthy choices will be challenging at first, but well worth the effort in the end. You need to choose what habits are most important to you and then promise yourself that you will stick to them. The best results are realized with consistency.

As you begin the score sheets for Week One, focus on the Healthy Habits and on the exercise goals. Don't worry about what habits lie ahead or whether your hunger levels change with the changes in your exercise routine. But always keep in mind the nutritional information you learned, and earn as many points as you can.

Steps to Success

There's a lot of information to absorb here, but if you take it one step at a time, you'll be amazed that such small changes can have such a big impact. When in doubt, just refer to these steps to success:

1. Exercise 5 days per week in the heart rate zones that are right for you.

2. Complete the Healthy Habits and activity score sheets every single day.

3. Total up your Healthy Habits points and your activity minutes at the end of each week.

4. Repeat your measurements at Week Four and record all new measurements.

5. Determine whether you need to follow the same exercise program or move up to the next level.

6. Continue to exercise 5 days per week in the heart rate zones that are right for you. Complete the Healthy Habits and activity score sheets every single day and add up your totals every week.

7. Repeat step 4 and record all of the final measurements.

8. Celebrate your success—reward yourself!

Healthy Habits 1-2

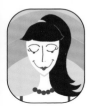

Welcome to Week One of the Spinning® 8-Week Weight Loss Program. Get ready to start feeling great about your nutritional habits and your active lifestyle. Week One will introduce you to some Healthy Habits that will be a simple yet vital element of this program.

Healthy Habit #1 - Stay between a 3 and a 6 on the hunger-satiety scale (20 points)

The first Healthy Habit involves using the hunger-satiety scale. The scale uses numbers from 1-10, which will help you to quantify the extent of your hunger and fullness throughout the day. It is OK to let yourself become hungry. In fact, hunger is the natural physiological mechanism that signals you to eat. The problem is, if you get too hungry and you allow yourself to reach numbers 1 and 2 on the scale, then you greatly increase the chance that you will overeat to the point that you reach a 7-10 on the scale. When you overeat, you impede your weight loss success. Overeating also comes with feelings of guilt, which are usually followed by over-restriction. During Week One, you need to break the starving-binging cycle and get back in tune with your natural hunger and satiety signals. Your body will let you know what you need. You just need to train yourself to listen and respond.

> Habitual snacking impedes weight loss success, but healthful snacking can do a great deal to prevent overeating.

10 = Stuffed to the point of feeling sick, in a food coma
9 = Very uncomfortably full, need to loosen your belt
8 = Uncomfortably full, feel stuffed
7 = Very full, feel as if you have overeaten
6 = Comfortably full, satisfied
5 = Neutral, neither hungry nor full
4 = Beginning signals of hunger
3 = Hungry, ready to eat
2 = Very hungry, unable to concentrate
1 = Starving, dizzy, irritable

How to do it:

1. Set a goal of eating at least three meals per day, evenly spaced apart (approximately 4 hours between meals).

2. Include healthy snacks in between meals if necessary. Keep some healthy snacks in your purse or briefcase, at the office and in your glove compartment. Habitual snacking impedes weight loss success, but healthful snacking can do a great deal to prevent overeating. However, you should try not to snack after dinner.

3. Try these healthy snacks: fruit, pre-cut raw vegetables, energy bars that DO NOT contain hydrogenated fats, yogurt, hummus and pita bread, natural peanut butter on whole-grain toast and whole-grain, low-sugar cereal (dry or with skim milk).

4. If you made a mistake and find yourself "starving," try the following tips to help prevent overeating:
   • Drink a large glass of water before eating.
   • Eat a little bit at a time, get up and do a task, then come back to eating. If you sit down and start shoveling in food, you will overeat. If you break up your eating, you will give your body more time to realize fullness.

5. Try not to eat while you are doing other things such as watching TV or driving. "Distracted eating" tends to make us lose awareness of how much we are eating. When this happens, we risk eating past the point of fullness.

6. When you are at home, try to eat only if you are sitting at the kitchen table.

7. Use smaller glasses and dishes. If it looks like you are getting more food, then you may eat less.

8. Eat slowly. Engaging in a conversation can help to slow your eating pace. So can setting down your utensils inbetween bites.

Motivation Tip:
Set yourself up for success. Being successful at reaching your goals takes more than just going through the motions. You have to set yourself up for acheivement instead of setting yourself up for failure. Get rid of things that might cause you to undermine your goals. If you still have junk food in your cabinet or baggy pants in your closet, then you are tempting yourself to break your fitness resolution. Align your environment with your goals, and watch as success comes to you more easily.

Exercise: Think about your daily routine and jot down some of the times and situations that tend to make you either extremely hungry, or uncomfortably full. Then think of ways to avoid those situations. For example, if you know that every time you work late you feel famished by the time you get home, you might want to keep some healthy leftovers at the office so you can still eat on time even when you can't get home for dinner.

_____

_____

_____

_____

_____

_____

_____

_____

_____

_____

_____

_____

_____

_____

_____

_____

Healthy Habit #2 - Drink at least 64 ounces of water per day (30 points)

Water is one of the closest things we have to a "magic bullet" that facilitates weight loss. You can drink plain water or seltzer water without sugar or any artificial sweeteners. Diet drinks and caffeine-containing beverages do NOT count toward your water goal.

Benefits:
- Water contains no calories. If you replace soda, diet drinks, fruit drinks and excess juice with water, you are bound to decrease your caloric intake and take a step closer to losing weight.
- Helps your body metabolize fat more efficiently.
- Prevents dehydration.
- Alleviates water retention, prevents bloating.
- Improves complexion.
- Decreases the chance that you will mistake hunger for thirst.
- Helps you to feel more energetic.

How to do it:
1. Drink a large glass of water when you wake up.
2. Have a second before you eat breakfast.
3. Drink one in the middle of the morning.
4. Have another before lunch.
5. Drink one in the afternoon.
6. Have another before dinner.
7 Drink one after dinner.
8. Drink enough water each day so that your urine is pale yellow.
9. Make sure to take a water bottle with you and drink it during ALL exercise sessions–not just Spinning® Program workouts. Note: A typical water bottle holds 24 ounces (3 cups).

Motivation Tip:
Keep your goal in sight (literally). Visual reinforcements are an effective tool in reminding you of what you aim to accomplish. Keep your goal in the forefront of your mind by posting a magazine clipping of a professional athlete or someone else you admire or want to look like on your refrigerator or pantry door. Or write a Mantra and hang it on your refrigerator door, such as: "I am stronger than temptation," or simply: "I promise to make a healthy choice today."

Exercise: List all the non-water beverages that you typically drink during the day. Which ones could you easily replace with water?

_____

_____

_____

_____

_____

_____

_____

_____

_____

_____

_____

_____

_____

_____

_____

_____

Using these two habits, you can earn up to a total of 50 points per day. Be sure to mark all your points on your score sheet in the logbook.

Sample Exercise Schedule

Your goal in Week One, just like every week, is to complete three Spinning® rides and two other days of exercise activity. If you're riding on your own and not as part of a class, the Ease Into It ride profile in the Workouts section of this manual is the perfect way to start out. Be sure to have a heart rate monitor, and that you don't let your intensity go beyond your Endurance Energy Zone™.

For your other exercise activities, use this sample schedule or create your own. But be sure to mix up the activities for variety and for a well-rounded fitness routine.

For illustrations and instructions, see the Workouts section at the end of this manual.

Day 1	Spinning®
Day 2	Spinning®
Day 3	Yoga
Day 4	Rest or light walk
Day 5	Spinning®
Day 6	Resist-A-Ball®
Day 7	Rest or light walk

Healthy Habits 3-4

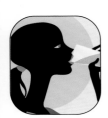

You've made it through Week One. You should be proud of yourself for any changes you made. Now you're on to Week Two, with two more habits to incorporate. Add these to your first two, keep exercising according to your plan, and do your best!

Continue to focus on and earn points for keeping your hunger and satiety in check and drinking a minimum of 64 ounces of water per day.

Healthy Habit #3 - Eat a healthy breakfast (30 points)

Too many people start off the day by deciding that they are going to eat healthy. They start by drinking a cup of coffee and eating a piece of toast or 1/2 a banana. They somehow make it to lunch (probably from the caffeine buzz) and select a salad or a cup of soup for lunch. At this point, they are proud of themselves for eating so little, and overlook the fact that they have the onset of a hunger headache. At this point they are so hungry that they snack on anything and every-thing accessible while they are preparing dinner, eat dinner, then continue eating after dinner until they go to bed feeling guilty and way too stuffed. They wonder why they have an eating problem and decide to start the following day by skipping breakfast. Does this sound familiar? Eating a healthy breakfast can be one of the best things you can do to break this cycle.

> Live by the saying
>
> "Eat like a king or
>
> queen at breakfast,
>
> eat like a prince or
>
> princess at lunch
>
> and eat like a pauper
>
> at dinner."

Live by the saying "Eat like a king or queen at breakfast, eat like a prince or princess at lunch and eat like a pauper at dinner."

Benefits:

- Breakfast speeds up your metabolism. Skipping it can cause your basal meta-bolic rate to drop by 40%. You cannot afford to have this happen if weight loss is your goal.
- It will increase your nutrition.
- Eating breakfast will help you to make healthier food choices throughout the day.
- Your metabolism is quicker in the morning, so your body is going to be more effective at burning calories that you take in earlier in the day.

How to do it:

1. Try eating dinner earlier and/or not snacking after dinner so that you are actually hungry when you wake up.

2. Wake up early enough so that you have time to eat. This may just be setting the alarm 10-15 minutes earlier.

3. Eat more than one food item for breakfast. Include at least one good source of protein so that you feel more satisfied.

4. Healthy breakfast ideas include:
   - One bowl of high fiber, whole grain cereal, 2 tablespoons of raisins and 1 cup of skim milk
   - One cup of plain yogurt mixed with 1 cup of strawberries and 1 slice of whole grain toast
   - One raisin bran English muffin, 2 tablespoons of natural peanut butter, 1 sliced banana

Motivation Tip:
Learn to overcome excuses. The mind is a powerful justifier, and often, it tries to let us get away with things we shouldn't be doing. "I stuck to my diet all week, so I can cheat today." Or "It's [Thanksgiving/Christmas/someone's Birthday/Anniversary, etc.] so I can make an exception this time." Recognize these thoughts as excuses and dismiss them. If you can remain aware of your excuses, then you can overcome them.

Exercise: Go to your kitchen and inventory your healthy breakfast items. If you're not a breakfast eater, you probably won't find much. Make a list of the groceries you need to buy in order to make breakfast your daily kick-off to a healthy day.

_____

_____

_____

_____

_____

_____

_____

_____

_____

_____

_____

_____

_____

_____

_____

_____

_____

_____

Healthy Habit #4 - Do not snack after dinner (30 points)
Most after-dinner snacking is more habitual than a result of actual need. Also, going to bed slightly hungry will increase the chances that you will wake up hungry, eat breakfast, maintain a healthy metabolism and be able to make better food choices throughout the day.

How to do it:
1. Clean up the kitchen after dinner. Put all leftovers away so that food is out of sight.

2. Brush and floss your teeth. This will get rid of the taste of food and make you think twice before you eat again.

3. If you find that you want to eat, try drinking a glass of water instead.

4. Keep yourself busy. Start a project or get out of the house. Go for a walk.

5. Go to sleep earlier. You cannot eat when you are sleeping. Additionally, adequate sleep enables you to make better food choices and improves your metabolism!

Motivation Tip:
Make it fun. One of the biggest determining factors in reaching your goal is having fun in the process. Get a friend to attend Spinning® class with you, and your workouts will start to feel like a social event. Or challenge your friends to reach their weight loss goals with you. Weigh in each week and let the winner be treated to a meal at a healthy restaurant. Incorporating your goal into games and social activities will make reaching your goal feel more fun, and less of a chore.

Exercise: Check the television listings and make a list of only the shows that you really want to watch this week. If you limit your TV nights, you'll probably snack less.

_____

_____

_____

_____

_____

_____

_____

_____

_____

_____

_____

_____

_____

_____

_____

_____

_____

Using these four Healthy Habits, you can earn up to a total of 110 points per day! Be sure to mark all your points on your score sheet.

Sample Exercise Schedule

If you completed three Spinning® rides in Week One, you can expect to feel a bit stronger and more comfortable on the bike this week. Keep up the good work and try the 6 Pak ride profile for one of your Week Two Spinning rides.

The sample exercise schedule this week includes the same workouts as in Week One. See if you can hold those Yoga asanas just a little longer and breathe a little deeper. During your Resist-A-Ball® workout, try adding a few more reps (as long as you can maintain good form).

For illustrations and instructions, see the Workouts section at the end of this manual.

Day 1	Spinning®
Day 2	Spinning®
Day 3	Resist-A-Ball®
Day 4	Rest or light walk
Day 5	Spinning®
Day 6	Yoga
Day 7	Rest or light walk

Healthy Habits 5-6

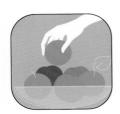

By now you're starting to learn to listen to your hunger cues, drink your water, cut out after-dinner snacking and eat breakfast. And don't forget your exercise goals. It's not so hard when your new habits require you to eat and drink more than you may have before. Here are two more.

Healthy Habit #5 - Eat at least six fruit and vegetable servings per day, excluding juice (30 points)

Benefits:
- Fruit and vegetables, even starchy vegetables, are low in calories.
- They are high in fiber.
- Since fruits and vegetables have a high water content, they may do more for satiety and weight control than their lighter, higher-fat counter parts.
- Replacing higher calorie foods with fruits and vegetables is a great calorie-reducing strategy. Eating lower calorie foods before a meal will help you to fill up faster and will leave less room for higher-calorie foods.
- Choosing to eat more fruits and vegetables will decrease your consumption of high fat, high sugar, highly processed foods.

How to do it:

1. Plan ahead. Eat a minimum of two fruit/vegetable servings at each meal.

2. Grocery shop frequently and make sure your kitchen is well stocked with fruits and vegetables.

3. When you get back from the grocery store wash, peel and prepare fruits and vegetables so that they are convenient to eat.

4. Make a fruit salad and squeeze in lemon juice to keep it fresh longer.

5. Make a smoothie or exercise recovery drink by mixing frozen fruit and yogurt or skim milk. Juice does not count towards this goal because you are not consuming the whole fruit. If you put fruit into a blender that is different because you will retain the fiber.

6. Keep frozen vegetables on hand so you do not have to worry about running out.

Motivation Tip:
Set up a rewards system. If you stick to your Healthy Habits for the week, treat yourself to a new book. When you lose your first 10 lbs., buy yourself a new outfit. If you set up rewards for reaching small, achievable milestones on the way to your goal, you won't want to get off track!

Exercise: Review the Nutrition 101 section in this manual and select the fruits and vegetables that you want to include in your diet. Then make a list of your choices, along with the serving sizes for each one. Example: 1/2 banana, 15 small grapes.

_____

_____

_____

_____

_____

_____

_____

_____

_____

_____

_____

_____

_____

_____

_____

_____

_____

_____

_____

_____

_____

Healthy Habit #6 - Do not eat any sweets or drink any alcoholic beverages (40 points)

Many sweets and alcoholic beverages can significantly add to your total daily caloric intake. Reducing the intake of these foods can dramatically contribute to creating a calorie deficit.

Foods included in this category are soda, fruit drinks, "diet" desserts, "diet" beverages, Jell-O®, pudding, frozen yogurt, Frappucinos®, cookies, cake, muffins, pie, ice cream, candy, chocolates, pastries, Pop-Tarts®, etc. Anything sugary, high in calories and without much nutrition counts as a sweet. Diet desserts are included in this category because many of them have fake sweeteners, preservatives, hydrogenated fats and unrecognizable ingredients.

Alcohol should be limited because it is almost as high in calories as fat, slows your metabolism, is dehydrating, increases the chance that you may overeat and may make you feel sluggish the next day.

How to do it:

1. Do not keep a bowl of candy on your desk at work or store tempting foods in your house.

2. If you really want a treat, make sure that getting it is an inconvenience. This will force you to think about whether or not you really need it.

3. Spend more time with your friends who are healthy eaters so that you will be positively influenced.

4. If you have to have a sweet, have a small portion. Check the serving size on the label (if it is available) and measure out the portion.

5. Keep in mind that some ice creams contain natural ingredients and have less added sugar, so their serving sizes contain fewer calories. Therefore, if you need a sweet, there are some better choices available.

Motivation Tip:
Maintain a positive outlook. Reaching your goal is going to take a lot of hard work. Don't focus on the things that you have to sacrifice to attain your goal. If you convince yourself that becoming healthy feels miserable because you don't get to indulge in your favorite sweets as often, then you are simply in need of a new perspective. Focus on the positive, and take care to rephrase any negative thoughts until they become positive. For example: "I hate that I have to cut back on sweets" can become: "I love that cutting back on sweets will make me look and feel great."

Exercise: Go through your kitchen right now and get rid of all the tempting sweets and alcoholic beverages that you want to cut out of your diet. Then, make a list of healthy desserts and beverages that you want to replace them with.

_____

_____

_____

_____

_____

_____

_____

_____

_____

_____

_____

_____

_____

_____

_____

_____

_____

Using these six Healthy Habits, you can now earn up to a total of 180 points per day! Be sure to mark all your points on your score sheet.

Sample Exercise Schedule

By now, you have completed enough Spinning® rides with consistency that you're likely to feel stronger and more powerful on the bike. Enjoy that feeling, but don't push too hard. Remember that you still need to watch your heart rate monitor. The Fat Burning Blast ride profile will keep you in the zone where you're training your body to burn fat for fuel.

The sample exercise schedule this week incorporates a mat workout that will really challenge your core! Be sure to follow the directions carefully for safe alignment and technique.

Day 1	Spinning®
Day 2	Mat Core Challenge
Day 3	Spinning®
Day 4	Rest or light walk
Day 5	Yoga
Day 6	Spinning®
Day 7	Rest or light walk

Healthy Habits 7-8

Congratulations! You are coming to the halfway point. Once you learn all these habits, you'll have another four weeks to practice them. By the end, they'll just be part of your regular routine. This week is also your opportunity to re-take your measurements and see all the progress you've made. Keep it up!

Healthy Habit #7 - Avoid consuming any hydrogenated and partially hydrogenated fats (40 points)

Benefits:
By eliminating consumption of hydrogenated fats, you will improve the quality of your diet, not burden your body with having to process hard-to-digest fats and will feel better. If you maintain this change beyond the Spinning® 8-Week Weight Loss Program, you will greatly reduce your risk of developing many of the most common diseases (high blood pressure, diabetes, obesity, heart disease and arthritis).

This one is the most challenging of the Habits, yet worth the effort, as it may be the most effective catalyst for change.

How to do it:

1. Avoid deep-fried foods.

2. Avoid "breaded" foods.

3. Avoid margarine and tub spreads.

4. Read the labels of all the food items you buy and avoid buying anything with the words "hydrogenated," "trans-fatty acids," "partially hydrogenated fats" and "shortening" listed in the ingredient category.

5. Prepare your own food as much as possible.

6. Limit the purchase of convenience foods.

7. Eat at restaurants less frequently. Most breads contain hydrogenated fats. Therefore, if you order a submarine sandwich or eat the rolls at a restaurant as an appetizer, you are probably consuming hydrogenated fats. Many diners and fast food restaurants use shortening or margarine for cooking, which means you would be consuming hydrogenated fats. You can only give yourself credit if you know for a fact that you did not consume hydrogenated fats.

8. If you do go out to eat, ask questions about how the food you are ordering is prepared.

9. Remember that fresh fruits and vegetables, frozen fruits and vegetables, nuts, seeds, dairy products, cheese, meat, fish, poultry and many whole grain foods DO NOT contain hydrogenated fats.

10. Try shopping in the "Natural Foods" aisle. There is a better chance that you will be able to find foods with nonhydrogenated fat.

11. Make sure that you read labels before buying cereals, crackers, chips, "reduced fat" foods, breads and snack foods.

Motivation Tip:
Take pride in your accomplishments, no matter how small. Every small step is bringing you closer to your goal. So try to keep track of your accomplishments, step-by-step, over time. Quantifying the number of pounds you are shedding, the number of inches you are losing and the decline in your percentage of body fat are all great ways to measure your success. Look back at your old measurements and notice the changes you have made so far! The numbers will empower you. And it only gets better from here.

Exercise: Think back to all the meals and snacks you've eaten over the past 2-3 days. List all the items you've eaten that contain hydrogenated and partially hydrogenated fats.

_____

_____

_____

_____

_____

_____

_____

_____

_____

_____

_____

_____

_____

_____

_____

_____

_____

_____

_____

_____

_____

Healthy Habit #8 - Avoid unnecessarily adding fat to food (20 points)

Benefits:
If you add less fat to foods, you will eat fewer calories and lose more weight. Most people eat adequate amounts of fat just through consuming meats, fish, poultry, cheeses, dairy products and nuts.

How to do it:
1. If you choose to use one of the healthy fats such as olive, canola or peanut oil when cooking, you will not lose points.

2. Avoid using margarine and "tub" spreads. Do not buy them. Do not keep them in the house. Virtually all of them contain hydrogenated fats.

3. Add a little olive oil and balsamic vinegar to salads.

4. Add a small amount of natural peanut, almond or apple butter to bread or toast instead of pure fats like cream cheese and butter.

5. Dip raw vegetables into hummus or salsa instead of creamy dips.

6. Don't order or cook deep-fried foods.

Motivation Tip:
Break your goal into mini-goals. If your goal is to lose 50 pounds, then it is easy to get frustrated when you see the pounds dropping off only 1 or 2 at a time. But if you create mini-goals, you can be proud of each small victory. Instead of saying: "I need to lose 50 pounds," say: "I want to lose just 1-2 lbs. per week through regular diet and exercise." At this rate, it would only take you 6-12 months to reach your overall weight loss goal!

Exercise: Make a grocery list of the items you need to buy to make sure you have healthy, low fat dips and dressings on hand when you need them.

_____

_____

_____

_____

_____

Congratulations! You have now learned all 8 Healthy Habits. Take a moment to review them now:

Healthy Habit #1 - Stay between a 3 and a 6 on the hunger-satiety scale.

Healthy Habit #2 - Drink at least 64 ounces of water per day.

Healthy Habit #3 - Eat a healthy breakfast.

Healthy Habit #4 - Do not snack after dinner.

Healthy Habit #5 - Eat at least six fruit and vegetable servings per day, excluding juice.

Healthy Habit #6 - Avoid or limit the intake of sweets and alcoholic beverages.

Healthy Habit #7 - Avoid consuming any hydrogenated and partially hydrogenated fats.

Healthy Habit #8 - Avoid unnecessarily adding fat to food.

Now that you have incorporated all eight Healthy Habits, you can earn up to a total of 240 points per day. You will continue to work on earning points for the remaining four weeks. Be sure to keep marking all your points on your score sheet. Remember that you start each day with "0" and accumulate points throughout the day.

Sample Exercise Schedule

You're halfway through the program, and it's time for your mid-point fitness measurements. That means you'll be going through another anaerobic threshold test, and you might see the number increase. If you do, congratulations. That indicates an improvement in your cardio respiratory fitness, and you can increase the challenge of your Spinning® rides with the Ride Strong profile. If your fitness test doesn't show an improvement, don't be discouraged. Three weeks is a good start toward your fitness level, but it may take another week or so to see a difference in your test results. Remember that if your anaerobic threshold and resting heart rate do change, you'll need to find your new Energy Zone™ heart rates on the Energy Zone charts.

The sample exercise schedule this week incorporates the same workouts you have learned in weeks 1-3. Remember, for an added challenge, you can always do more reps or add more time to your Spinning rides.

For illustrations and instructions, see the Workouts section at the end of this manual.

Day 1	Spinning®
Day 2	Mat Core Challenge
Day 3	Spinning®
Day 4	Rest or light walk
Day 5	Resist-A-Ball®
Day 6	Spinning®
Day 7	Rest or light walk

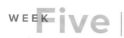

Congratulations! You are halfway through the 8-Week Program, and you have learned all 8 Healthy Habits. Your goal now is to continue to exercise and practice the habits each day. Think of this week as a fresh beginning. Don't worry if you feel you haven't done your best on the habits up to this point. Be proud of yourself for making it this far, and recognize that you've learned a lot. Now that you have some familiarity with the Healthy Habits and the score sheets routine, you'll find that the next four weeks will get easier and easier.

Exercise: Reflect back on the past four weeks. What has been the most challenging for you? What has been the most rewarding? Take some time to journal about the hurdles you've overcome and the lifestyle changes you've made.

_____

_____

_____

_____

_____

_____

_____

_____

_____

_____

_____

_____

Exercise: Refer to the Healthy Habits summary at the end of this section. Then, list all of the ways you have practiced these habits throughout the day. If you have not practiced these habits today, write about what you can do differently tomorrow to make them a part of your daily routine.

_____

_____

_____

_____

_____

_____

_____

_____

_____

_____

_____

_____

_____

_____

_____

_____

_____

_____

_____

_____

TEST YOUR KNOWLEDGE

1. Starving helps to accelerate weight loss and contributes to long-term success.　　T　F

2. Using smaller plates, glasses, bowls and utensils can contribute to consuming smaller portions.　　T　F

3. Designating specific eating areas (away from the T.V.) can help you to consume fewer calories.　　T　F

4. To achieve drinking 64-ounces of water per day, you should try to drink water only during mealtimes.　　T　F

5. Eating breakfast can help boost your metabolism.　　T　F

6. Eating light later in the day will increase your chances of being hungry for breakfast the next day.　　T　F

7. Getting the taste of food out of your mouth by brushing, flossing and using mouth wash can reduce the urge to eat after dinner.　　T　F

8. Even starchy vegetables may contribute to your daily fruit and vegetable servings goal.　　T　F

9. Frozen vegetables are a viable option if you are concerned about running out of fresh produce.　　T　F

10. Reducing overall intake of sweets and alcohol, even if you cannot eliminate these foods from your diet, can still contribute to weight loss success.　　T　F

11. "Diet" desserts don't count as sweets.　　T　F

12. Many different margarines that are marketed as being healthier than butter can still contain hydrogenated fats.　　T　F

13. If a food has no trans fats, then it does not contain hydrogenated fats.　　T　F

14. When you go out to eat, asking the server more about how food is prepared can be helpful in making healthier choices and reducing hydrogenated fat intake.　　T　F

15. Adding fat to foods will ensure that you will be more satisfied after meals, which can lead to reduced calorie intake.　　T　F

Answers: 1. F, 2. T, 3. T, 4. F, 5. T, 6. T, 7. T, 8. T, 9. T, 10. T, 11. F, 12. T, 13. F, 14. T, 15. F

Healthy Habits Summary

Healthy Habit #1 - Stay between a 3 and a 6 on the hunger-satiety scale.

Healthy Habit #2 - Drink at least 64 ounces of water per day.

Healthy Habit #3 - Eat a healthy breakfast.

Healthy Habit #4 - Do not snack after dinner.

Healthy Habit #5 - Eat at least six fruit and vegetable servings per day, excluding juice.

Healthy Habit #6 - Avoid or limit the intake of sweets and alcoholic beverages.

Healthy Habit #7 - Avoid consuming any hydrogenated and partially hydrogenated fats.

Healthy Habit #8 - Avoid unnecessarily adding fat to food.

Sample Exercise Schedule

If you're ready for a really challenging Spinning® ride, you'll love Peak Fitness Journey. Remember, recovery time is critical to your success in any fitness program, so be sure to thoroughly cool down at the end of an intense ride, and let your Yoga day be a light workout.

Day 1	Spinning®
Day 2	Mat Core Challenge
Day 3	Spinning®
Day 4	Rest or light walk
Day 5	Resist-A-Ball®
Day 6	Spinning®
Day 7	Rest or light walk

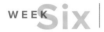
WEEK Six

You've now practiced all 8 Healthy Habits for two full weeks. Hopefully, the routine is getting easier. Perhaps you don't even have to think about it much. If so, this is a good time to focus more on your Spinning® rides. Review your Activity Log and make sure you're spending enough time in the Endurance Energy Zone™—the most important zone for building an aerobic base and burning fat. Turn to the Energy Zone section of this manual to review the Endurance Energy Zone benefits.

Exercise: Jot down 2-3 personal fitness and health goals you want to achieve through training in the Endurance Energy Zone.

_____

_____

_____

_____

_____

_____

_____

_____

_____

_____

_____

_____

_____

_____

_____

Exercise: Refer to the Spinning ride profiles located in the "Workouts" section of this manual. Browse the profiles provided and pick one that best fits your interests. (For example: If you are interested in increasing the amount of time spent in the Endurance Energy Zone, you might pick the Fat Burning Blast profile, which features a 50-minute Endurance ride). Then, write about why you are drawn to that particular ride, and how you will fit it into your workout schedule for the week.

_____

_____

_____

_____

_____

_____

_____

_____

_____

_____

_____

_____

_____

_____

_____

_____

_____

TEST YOUR KNOWLEDGE

1. People who eat less frequently are less likely to be overweight.   T   F

2. If you follow the Healthy Habits in this program, then you should never be hungry.   T   F

3. Distracted eating refers to having a conversation with someone while eating dinner at the kitchen table.   T   F

4. Replacing calorie-containing beverages with water can contribute to calorie reduction and weight loss.   T   F

5. Consuming more water can help reduce the amount of food you eat.   T   F

6. A cup of coffee with cream is a healthy substitute for breakfast.   T   F

7. Including a source of protein at breakfast can make you feel more satisfied and less hungry in the hours directly following breakfast.   T   F

8. Most people who eat after dinner need those extra calories.   T   F

9. Getting involved in a project or going for a walk after dinner can take your mind off of food.   T   F

10. Consuming higher calorie foods helps you feel full faster, which can contribute to an overall reduction in your calorie intake.   T   F

11. Food that is high in water content can make you feel fuller, which can help you eat less.   T   F

12. Keeping a bowl of candy on your desk at work is a great exercise in strengthening your will power.   T   F

13. The way hydrogenated fats are processed can contribute to health problems including high cholesterol, weight gain and high blood pressure.   T   F

14. All foods that are advertised as fat-free or trans-fat free contain 0 grams of fat.   T   F

15. You should try tasting food first, before assuming that you need to add fat to it.   T   F

Answers: 1. F, 2. F, 3. F, 4. T, 5. T, 6. F, 7. T, 8. F, 9. T, 10. F, 11. T, 12. F, 13. T, 14. F, 15. T

Healthy Habits Summary

Healthy Habit #1 - Stay between a 3 and a 6 on the hunger-satiety scale.

Healthy Habit #2 - Drink at least 64 ounces of water per day.

Healthy Habit #3 - Eat a healthy breakfast.

Healthy Habit #4 - Do not snack after dinner.

Healthy Habit #5 - Eat at least six fruit and vegetable servings per day, excluding juice.

Healthy Habit #6 - Avoid or limit the intake of sweets and alcoholic beverages.

Healthy Habit #7 - Avoid consuming any hydrogenated and partially hydrogenated fats.

Healthy Habit #8 - Avoid unnecessarily adding fat to food.

Sample Exercise Schedule

Now that you've established a good base of consistency with exercise, try a Spinning® ride that's a little longer than usual. The Burn ride profile is a challenging 45-minute interval training workout. You may also want to increase the duration of your Mat Core Challenge workouts. Try repeating the entire exercise sequence twice!

Day 1	Spinning®
Day 2	Mat Core Challenge
Day 3	Resist-A-Ball®
Day 4	Rest or easy bike ride
Day 5	Spinning®
Day 6	Spinning®
Day 7	Rest

WEEK Seven |

You're almost done. Only two more weeks to go. This is the time to challenge yourself a bit more. Can you schedule in an extra exercise session or two? Can you climb those hills with a bit more resistance? Can you strive to set your personal record in weekly points in your Healthy Habits logbook? Whatever challenge you decide to take on, make it one that will give you a sense of accomplishment. Enjoy that feeling—you deserve it.

Exercise: Decide on one or more challenges for yourself and then list your goals for the week.

_____

_____

_____

_____

_____

_____

_____

_____

_____

_____

_____

_____

_____

_____

_____

_____

Exercise: Think about how good it would feel to achieve all of your weight loss goals. Understand that in these final weeks, you must push yourself to the limit to achieve them. What can you do now to ensure your overall success in the program? Where do you usually slip up? Be honest with yourself and write down a list of your weaknesses. Then write down several ways that you can overcome them, to prevent future slip ups.

_____

_____

_____

_____

_____

_____

_____

_____

_____

_____

_____

_____

_____

_____

_____

_____

_____

TEST YOUR KNOWLEDGE

1. Healthy snacking can contribute to long term weight loss success.　　T　F

2. Developing strategies that help you to eat more slowly will reduce your caloric intake.　　T　F

3. Drinking water before meals, with meals and between meals is recommended.　　T　F

4. Drinking diet soda or flavored water with artificial sweeteners counts toward your 64-ounce water goal.　　T　F

5. If you consume large amounts of food in the evening, it means that you probably did not eat enough healthful foods to satisfy you throughout the day.　　T　F

6. Over-consuming calories in the evening can lead to feeling 'full' and guilty the following morning, which may reduce your motivation to eat breakfast.　　T　F

7. Habits or routines can sometimes cause people to eat when they are not actually hungry.　　T　F

8. People who eat after dinner usually did not eat breakfast.　　T　F

9. Going to sleep earlier can steer you away from late-night snacking.　　T　F

10. Fiber from fruits and vegetables can help you feel full without providing extra calories that are in other foods.　　T　F

11. Choosing sweets that naturally contain fewer calories (less added sugars/less added fat) can help with weight loss.　　T　F

12. Making sweets and alcohol less accessible can backfire and lead to an obsession with these foods.　　T　F

13. Eliminating deep fried foods is an important strategy in reducing hydrogenated fat intake.　　T　F

14. Reading the ingredient label is the best way to identify the presence of hydrogenated fats in a food.　　T　F

15. Over time, you can adjust to enjoying foods without added fat.　　T　F

Answers: 1. T, 2. T, 3. T, 4. F, 5. T, 6. T, 7. T, 8. F, 9. T, 10. T, 11. T, 12. F, 13. T, 14. T, 15. T

Healthy Habits Summary

Healthy Habit #1 - Stay between a 3 and a 6 on the hunger-satiety scale.

Healthy Habit #2 - Drink at least 64 ounces of water per day.

Healthy Habit #3 - Eat a healthy breakfast.

Healthy Habit #4 - Do not snack after dinner.

Healthy Habit #5 - Eat at least six fruit and vegetable servings per day, excluding juice.

Healthy Habit #6 - Avoid or limit the intake of sweets and alcoholic beverages.

Healthy Habit #7 - Avoid consuming any hydrogenated and partially hydrogenated fats.

Healthy Habit #8 - Avoid unnecessarily adding fat to food.

Sample Exercise Schedule

This week, let your Spinning® rides motivate you to reach the goals you've set for yourself. There may be days when you don't feel like exercising, but remember that once you get on the bike, start pedaling and feel the music, the motivation will come from within. Try doing the Aerobic Loops and Ladders ride profile this week, to inspire you to climb to the top!

Day 1	Spinning®
Day 2	Mat Core Challenge
Day 3	Resist-A-Ball®
Day 4	Rest or easy bike ride
Day 5	Spinning®
Day 6	Spinning®
Day 7	Rest

This is it! The final week. Enjoy it, be proud and finish strong. But remember that the end of Week Eight is not the end of your new healthy lifestyle. You've learned a lot, you've grown and you've become a better you. And those changes can stay with you for a lifetime.

Exercise: Write yourself your own congratulatory letter. Don't be shy! Remind yourself of all the changes you've made in your life and the challenges you've overcome. Write down anything you want to acknowledge about your achievement.

_____

_____

_____

_____

_____

_____

_____

_____

_____

_____

_____

_____

_____

_____

_____

_____

_____

_____

Exercise: Now that you have made it to the final week of your Spinning weight loss journey, you have seen firsthand what determination and dedication can achieve. Besides weight loss, consider what other goals you might have for yourself. No matter the goal, you should now have the confidence you need to achieve it. Write about what else you want to do to improve your life. Then, write down the steps to achieve that goal, and empower yourself to do it!

_____

_____

_____

_____

_____

_____

_____

_____

_____

_____

_____

_____

_____

_____

_____

_____

_____

TEST YOUR KNOWLEDGE

1. Assessing how hungry you are before you eat can keep you from eating more than you are hungry for.   T   F

2. Developing strategies that help you to eat more slowly will increase your caloric intake.   T   F

3. Drinking more water can reduce the risk of becoming dehydrated during exercise and ultimately enhance performance.   T   F

4. Eating less for breakfast and more at dinner can lead to overall reduced calorie consumption.   T   F

5. Stocking your kitchen with healthy breakfast foods can contribute to eating more than you are hungry for at breakfast.   T   F

6. Storing food out of sight can help reduce the urge to eat.   T   F

7. Eating more fruits and vegetables will leave you less satisfied, driving you to eat more high-sugar, high-fat snack foods.   T   F

8. Fruits and vegetables are most effective in your diet when they are consumed to replace higher calorie foods.   T   F

9. Washing, cutting and preparing produce upon returning from the grocery store can help increase fruit and vegetable intake.   T   F

10. Alcohol is almost as high in calories as it is in fat.   T   F

11. Surrounding yourself with others that eat healthy can help to improve your own eating habits.   T   F

12. Partially hydrogenated and fully hydrogenated fats have gone through unnatural processing and both are to be avoided.   T   F

13. Avoiding hydrogenated fats can provide motivation to prepare more of your own food from scratch.   T   F

14. Natural nut butters, though they contain fat, also provide other nutrients like fiber and protein, which can make them a better choice than a pure fat like butter or margarine.   T   F

15. People consume enough fats from eating nuts, meats and cheeses without having to add extra fats (like margarine) to their food.   T   F

Answers: 1. T, 2. F, 3. T, 4. F, 5. F, 6. T, 7. F, 8. T, 9. T, 10. T, 11. T, 12. T, 13. T, 14. T, 15. T

Healthy Habits Summary

Healthy Habit #1 -   Stay between a 3 and a 6 on the hunger-satiety scale.

Healthy Habit #2 -   Drink at least 64 ounces of water per day.

Healthy Habit #3 -   Eat a healthy breakfast.

Healthy Habit #4 -   Do not snack after dinner.

Healthy Habit #5 -   Eat at least six fruit and vegetable servings per day, excluding juice.

Healthy Habit #6 -   Avoid or limit the intake of sweets and alcoholic beverages.

Healthy Habit #7 -   Avoid consuming any hydrogenated and partially hydrogenated fats.

Healthy Habit #8 -   Avoid unnecessarily adding fat to food.

Sample Exercise Schedule

Anaerobic Hills and Valleys is the most challenging Spinning® ride profile so far! Use the inspiration you've gained from this program to power you through it.

Day 1	Spinning®
Day 2	Mat Core Challenge (2x)
Day 3	Rest or easy bike ride
Day 4	Spinning®
Day 5	Yoga
Day 6	Spinning®
Day 7	Rest

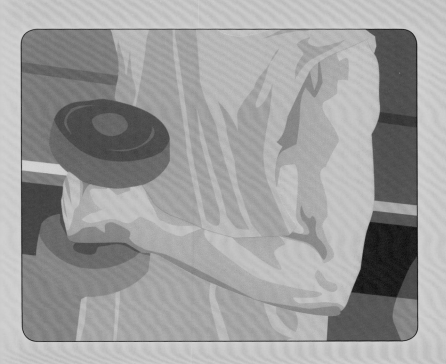

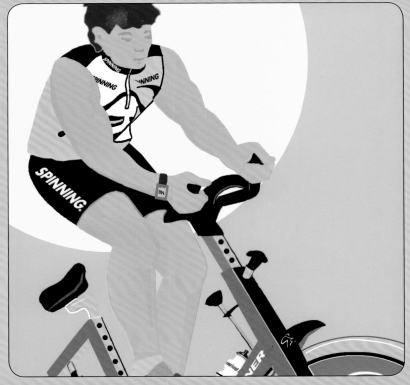

Workouts

In the Spinning® 8-Week Weight Loss Program, your goal is to complete three Spinning rides and two days of other exercise activities per week. You can use the sample workouts provided in this section to help meet those goals. Choose from 8 Spinning ride profiles (1 new profile for each week of the program), in addition to our Yoga, Resist-A-Ball® and Mat Core Challenge sample workouts.

For a wide selection of fitness balls and other equipment, visit www.spinning.com.

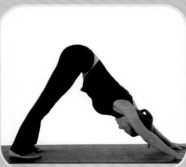

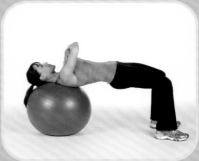

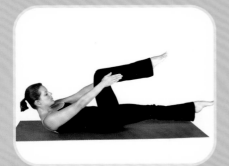

Ease Into It

CREATED BY	Meg McNeely
ENERGY ZONE™	**Endurance**
RIDE LENGTH	40 minutes
RIDE DESCRIPTION	Focus on increasing heart rate and controlling it as it slowly rises. Riding at a specifically dictated heart rate for a long period of time teaches a controlled way of stabilizing heart rate. You will achieve a deeper awareness of breath and mental discipline while increasing heart rate to reach 75% maximum heart rate (MHR) by the end of the journey.

Elapsed Time	Duration	Movement	Intensity	Cadence	Technique
0:00–5:00	5 min	Seated Flat	65% MHR	80–90 RPM	Warm up for 5–8 minutes and raise heart rate to about 65% MHR.
5:00–10:00	5 min	Seated Flat	65% MHR	80–110 RPM	Take time to clear the mind and master well-controlled breathing while getting rid of negative thoughts and worries. Focus on yourself for the next 40 minutes.
10:00–25:00	15 min	Seated Flat / Standing Flat	70% MHR	80–110 RPM	You can rise out of the saddle for 30 seconds at a time for Standing Flats. Use this time to practice pedal stroke fluidity. While adding only a few RPM at a time, notice how it affects the heart rate. Maintain 70% MHR. Next, play with the resistance and note how it also affects heart rate. Take this time also to perfect form and rediscover different breathing patterns and techniques.
25:00–35:00	10 min	Seated Climb	75% MHR	60–80 RPM	Again, 30-second bouts off the saddle are an option, but make sure heart rate stays at or below 75% MHR. Use core strength to support yourself. Combine strength and elegance while climbing.
35:00–40:00	5 min	Seated Flat		80–90 RPM	Cool down.

6 Pak

CREATED BY	Sherri Crilly
ENERGY ZONE™	**Endurance**
RIDE LENGTH	40 minutes
RIDE DESCRIPTION	This profile was created to help those who have a hard time sitting in the saddle for more than a few minutes at a time. It also gives you an opportunity to determine your preferred cadence in each movement.

Elapsed Time	Duration	Movement	Intensity	Cadence	Technique
0:00–5:00	5 min	Seated Flat	65% MHR	80–100 RPM	Warm up. Choose a comfortable cadence to get the legs rolling.
5:00–8:00	3 min	Seated Flat	75% MHR	80–100 RPM	Increase the resistance slightly so that you can maintain your preferred cadence while increasing your heart rate.
8:00–11:00	3 min	Standing Flat	80% MHR	70–90 RPM	Find your preferred cadence while standing, allowing your heart rate to increase to 80% MHR.
11:00–15:00	4 min	Seated Flat	75–80% MHR	90–100 RPM	Maintaining your preferred cadence, focus on pedal stroke drills as you gently increase the resistance.
15:00–17:00	2 min	Standing Flat	80% MHR	70–90 RPM	Maintain your gear as you drop cadence slightly.
17:00–23:00	6 min	Seated Climb	80% MHR	60–80 RPM	Control your heart rate while feeling light and rhythmic, and take time to adapt to this increased load.
23:00–28:00	5 min	Seated Climb	80% MHR	60–80 RPM	Maintaining your preferred cadence, gently add some gear, using breath to control your heart rate.
28:00–29:00	1 min	Standing Climb	80% MHR	60–80 RPM	Use this time to stretch your legs and get rid of any fatigue. Gently increase your RPM by 5-8.
29:00–33:00	4 min	Seated Flat	80% MHR	80–90 RPM	Release just enough gear to raise your cadence as you return back to a flat road.
33:00–35:00	2 min	Standing Flat	80% MHR	80–90 RPM	Focus on proper pedal stroke without allowing fatigue to set in.
35:00–37:00	2 min	Standing Flat	75% MHR	80–90 RPM	Enjoy what you have just accomplished! You just trained for muscular endurance and overload at the same time!
37:00–40:00	3 min	Seated Flat	65% MHR	90–100 RPM	Cool down as your energy revitalizes.

Fat Burning Blast

CREATED BY	Jennifer Ward
ENERGY ZONE™	**Endurance**
RIDE LENGTH	50 minutes
RIDE DESCRIPTION	This ride is structured in a pyramid format with Seated Flat and Seated Climb movements. The goal is to increase aerobic fitness and the body's ability to burn fat more efficiently. As you progress up the pyramid, each Seated Flat will become shorter as each Seated Climb becomes longer, and vice versa on the way down.

Elapsed Time	Duration	Movement	Intensity	Cadence	Technique
0:00–14:00	14 min	Seated Flat	65% MHR	80–90 RPM	Move through single-leg focus drills for 5 minutes of the warm-up. Alternate focus for 30 seconds on each leg.
14:00–15:00	1 min	Seated Climb	75% MHR	60–80 RPM	Hold the Seated Climb for 1 minute. As you progress up the pyramid, each Seated Climb will become longer.
15:00–15:30	30 sec	Standing Flat	75% MHR	80–110 RPM	Use techniques practiced in the single-leg focus drills to maintain a steady heart rate and perfect form.
15:30–21:00	5 min 30 sec		65–75% MHR	80–110 RPM	Repeat the series. Hold the Seated Flat for 3 minutes, the Seated Climb for 2, and the Standing Flat for 30 seconds.
21:00–26:30	5 min 30 sec		65–75% MHR	80–110 RPM	Repeat again. **This time:** Hold the Seated Flat for 2 minutes, the Seated Climb for 3 minutes, and the Standing Flat for 30 seconds.
26:30–32:00	5 min 30 sec	Standing Flat	65–75% MHR	80–100 RPM	Use techniques practiced in the single-leg focus drills to maintain a steady heart rate and perfect form.
32:00–37:30	5 min 30 sec		65–75% MHR	80–110 RPM	Repeat again. Seated Flat: 1 min; Seated Climb: 4 min; Standing Flat: 30 seconds.
37:30–43:00	5 min 30 sec		65–75% MHR	80–110 RPM	Last repeat. Seated Flat: 3 min; Seated Climb: 2 min; Standing Flat: 30 seconds
43:00–50:00	7 min	Seated Flat	65% MHR	80–110 RPM	Cool down.

Ride Strong

CREATED BY	Donna Minotti
ENERGY ZONE™	**Strength**
RIDE LENGTH	55 minutes
RIDE DESCRIPTION	The first portion of this profile repeats a set of movements in increasing duration for each interval. For the second portion, you'll repeat 2-minute intervals with 1 minute of work and 1 minute of recovery.

Elapsed Time	Duration	Movement	Intensity	Cadence	Technique
0:00–5:00	5 min	Seated Flat	65% MHR		Warm up.
5:00–8:00	3 min	Seated Climb, Jumps on a Hill, Standing Climb	75% MHR	60–80 RPM	30 sec. for each movement: Seated Climb: 30 sec. Jumps: 30 sec. Standing Climb: 30 sec. Repeat.
8:00–14:00	6 min	Seated Climb, Jumps on a Hill, Standing Climb	80% MHR	60–80 RPM	1 minute for each movement. Repeat.
14:00–23:00	9 min	Seated Climb, Jumps on a Hill, Standing Climb	80% MHR	60–80 RPM	90 sec. for each movement. Repeat.
23:00–35:00	12 min	Seated Climb, Jumps on a Hill, Standing Climb	80% MHR	60–80 RPM	2 minutes for each movement. Repeat.
35:00–37:00	2 min	Standing Climb, Running with Resistance, Seated Flat	80–85% MHR	60–80 RPM	Standing Climb: 45 sec. Running with Resistance: 15 sec. 1 minute recovery in Seated Flat.
37:00–51:00	14 min		80–85% MHR	60–80 RPM	Repeat minutes 35:00–37:00 seven times.
51:00–55:00	4 min	Seated Flat	65% MHR	80–110 RPM	Cool down and stretch.

CREATED BY	Jennifer Ward
ENERGY ZONE™	**Interval**
RIDE LENGTH	40 minutes
RIDE DESCRIPTION	This ride is designed to get you on the road to peak fitness and performance, by mixing anaerobic work with recovery periods. This profile was inspired by an outdoor ride, and includes two major climbing sections that will help you improve your power and acceleration.

Elapsed Time	Duration	Movement	Intensity	Cadence	Technique
0:00–7:00	7 min	Seated Flat	65% MHR	80–90 RPM	Warm up for 7 minutes and raise your heart rate to about 65% maximum heart rate (MHR).
7:00–8:00	1 min	Seated Flat	70% MHR	90–100 RPM	Increase intensity through speed and resistance.
8:00–8:30	30 sec	Standing Climb	80% MHR	60–80 RPM	Increase resistance and accelerate uphill for 30 seconds.
8:30–10:00	1 min 30 sec		70-80% MHR	80–100 RPM	Repeat minutes 7:00–8:30.
10:00–13:00	3 min	Seated Flat	75% MHR	80–110 RPM	Increase resistance every minute until you reach the base of a hill.
13:00–15:30	2 min 30 sec	Seated Climb	75-85% MHR	60–80 RPM	Slightly increase resistance every 30 seconds while working to maintain a cadence between 60–80 RPM.
15:30–18:30	3 min	Standing Climb	85-92% MHR	60–80 RPM	Hill steepness increases. Shift position to a challenging Standing Climb.
18:30–19:30	1 min	Seated Flat	65-70% MHR	90–110 RPM	Increase the resistance. Stay on the flat, but make the transition into a "working" flat.
19:30–20:30	1 min	Jumps	75-85% MHR	80–90 RPM	Add extra effort on the Jumps. Accelerate slightly to increase the intensity.
20:30–24:30	4 min		65-85% MHR	80–110 RPM	Repeat minutes 18:30–20:30 twice.
24:30–25:30	1 min	Seated Flat	65-70% MHR	90–100 RPM	Ride easy on the flat.
25:30–30:00	4 min 30 sec	Standing Climb	85-92% MHR	60 RPM	Ride with the hardest resistance possible.
30:00–34:00	4 min	Seated Flat	60-65% MHR	90–100 RPM	Recover in the saddle as you ride down the backside of that second big hill.
34:00–40:00	6 min	Seated Flat	75-80% MHR	80–90 RPM	Ride easy on the flat and cool down. You did it!

Burn

CREATED BY	Jennifer Ward
ENERGY ZONE™	**Interval**
RIDE LENGTH	45 minutes
RIDE DESCRIPTION	Although these intense intervals decrease in length, you will have to ramp up the intensity with each one to reach the target heart rate (HR). Find a balance of gauging resistance, ramping up heart rate and sustaining an impressive performance throughout the interval. This is vital if you are performance-focused or have demonstrated consistency in aerobic fitness.

Elapsed Time	Duration	Movement	Intensity	Cadence	Technique
0:00–10:00	10 min	Seated Flat	55–65% MHR	80–110 RPM	Perform muscle-focus drills on the quads, glutes, hamstrings, hip flexors. Spend 2 minutes focusing on each of the muscle groups with a bit more force to help identify what role each group plays in the pedal stroke.
10:00–12:00	2 min	Standing Flat	65–75% MHR	80–110 RPM	Use the Standing Flat to elevate heart rate. Continue to effectively utilize all muscles involved in driving the pedals.
12:00–13:00	1 min	Seated Climb	75–80% MHR	60–80 RPM	Use the climb to elevate heart rate to the aerobic ceiling.
13:00–14:00	1 min	Seated Flat	65% MHR	80–110 RPM	Use the recovery to recharge and prepare for the interval.
14:00–20:00	6 min	Standing Climb / Sprints on a Hill	85–92% MHR	60–80 RPM	Drive the resistance and heart rate up. Charge up the hill. Pick up the pace and do sprints on a hill for the last 10 seconds, working beyond your lactate threshold.
20:00–24:00	4 min	Seated Flat	60–65% MHR	80–100 RPM	Ride easy and recover.
24:00–34:00	10 min				Repeat minutes 14:00–24:00.
34:00–40:00	6 min	Standing Climb / Sprints on a Hill	85–92% MHR	60–80 RPM	One final work effort, this time for a short duration. Drive the resistance and heart rate up. Charge up the hill one last time. Pick up the pace and do sprints on a hill for the last 10 seconds.
40:00–45:00	5 min	Seated Flat	55–65% MHR	80–100 RPM	Cool down.

Aerobic Loops and Ladders

SPINNING

CREATED BY	Sabrina Fairchild
ENERGY ZONE™	**Interval**
RIDE LENGTH	40 minutes
RIDE DESCRIPTION	A ladder of intervals starting with a 3-minute work segment and eventually increasing to 4 minutes of work, on varied terrain.

Elapsed Time	Duration	Movement	Intensity	Cadence	Technique
0:00–6:00	6 min	Seated Flat	50–65% MHR	80–100 RPM	Bring your awareness to your breath and discover how using your breath for recovery will improve your comfort and performance.
6:00–9:00	3 min	Standing Flat	75% MHR	80–90 RPM	Adjust resistance/gear or cadence to elevate HR for 3 minutes.
9:00–10:00	1 min	Seated Flat	65% MHR	80–90 RPM	For recovery, decrease gear and sit for 1 minute.
10:00–13:00	3 min	Jumps	75% MHR	80–100 RPM	Add gear for Jumps and choose your own pace for 3 minutes.
13:00–14:00	1 min	Seated Flat	65% MHR	70–90 RPM	For recovery, decrease gear and stay in the saddle for 1 minute.
14:00–17:00	3 min	Seated Climb	75–80% MHR	60–70 RPM	Add moderate to heavy resistance for 3 minutes.
17:00–18:00	1 min	Seated Flat	65% MHR	80–90 RPM	For 1 minute of recovery, reduce gear and increase cadence while seated.
18:00–22:00	4 min	Standing Flat	75% MHR	80–90 RPM	Same as first set. Add gear and stand for 4 minutes.
22:00–23:00	1 min	Seated Flat	65% MHR	80–90 RPM	Reduce gear for seated recovery for 1 minute.
23:00–27:00	4 min	Jumps	75–80% MHR	80–100 RPM	Add gear for Jumps and choose your own pace for 4 minutes.
27:00–28:00	1 min	Seated Flat	65% MHR	80–90 RPM	Reduce gear and be seated for a 1-minute recovery. Hydrate.
28:00–32:00	4 min	Seated Climb	75–80% MHR	60–70 RPM	Add heavy gear for a 4-minute hill. Focus on pushing forward between 10 o'clock and 2 o'clock on the pedal stroke. Work hard. This is your last work interval.
32:00–40:00	8 min	Seated Flat	50–65% MHR	80–90 RPM	Recover and cool down.

Anaerobic Hills and Valleys

CREATED BY	Sabrina Fairchild
ENERGY ZONE™	**Interval**
RIDE LENGTH	40 minutes
RIDE DESCRIPTION	This ride features hills and valleys for anaerobic training of up to 92% of your maximum heart rate (MHR).

Elapsed Time	Duration	Movement	Intensity	Cadence	Technique
0:00–4:00	4 min	Seated Flat	50–65% MHR	90–100 RPM	This warm-up has three stages to prepare you for the grueling session ahead. **Stage 1:** Start slow and ration your energy.
4:00–9:00	5 min	Standing Flat	60–70% MHR	80–100 RPM	**Stage 2:** Elevate your heart rate (HR) while preparing your muscles for more standing work. Use moderate resistance.
9:00–13:00	4 min	Jumps	70–80% MHR	80–100 RPM	**Stage 3:** Transition into Jumps. Pace yourself to increase your target heart rate zone.
13:00–15:00	2 min	Standing Flat	85–92% MHR	90–108 RPM	Increase your cadence to gradually reach your target HR. The goal is to reach at least 85% MHR.
15:00–19:00	4 min	Seated Flat	70–80% MHR	90–108 RPM	Increase your cadence until your target heart rate has been achieved.
19:00–21:00	2 min	Standing Climb	85–92% MHR	70–80 RPM	Increase resistance again and transition into a Standing Climb in HP 3.
21:00–23:00	2 min	Seated Flat	65% MHR	80–90 RPM	Reduce resistance to allow for deep breathing. Hydrate.
23:00–25:00	2 min	Seated Flat	70–75% MHR	90–108 RPM	Increase resistance first, and then increase cadence. Imagine a strong wind coming up against you.
25:00–27:00	2 min	Standing Flat	75–85% MHR	90–108 RPM	Add gear and gradually elevate HR into your target zone in 5–10 beats per minute.
27:00–30:00	3 min	Seated Flat	65% MHR	80–90 RPM	Reduce gear and cadence. The key here is to maintain 65% MHR.
30:00–32:00	2 min	Standing Climb	85% MHR	60–70 RPM	Add heavy resistance.
32:00–34:00	2 min	Standing Climb	85–92% MHR	70–80 RPM	Increase cadence and resistance if necessary to achieve anaerobic HR range.
34:00–40:00	6 min	Seated Flat	50–65% MHR	80–90 RPM	Decrease gear to lower your HR to 50% and complete the cool-down.

Yoga Asana Sequence Workout

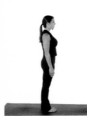

Mountain Pose
Stand with feet hip distance apart. Distribute weight evenly across the bottom of both feet.

Standing Forward Bend
Hinge from the hips and fold forward, bringing your forehead to meet your knees while keeping your legs straight.

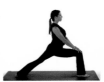

Warrior
Bring one foot forward in a lunge; back leg straight. Lift the chest and bring the hands above the knee.

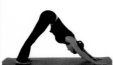

Downward Facing Dog
Straighten the legs and lift the tailbone toward the ceiling. Keep weight evenly distributed between hands and feet.

Warrior
Bring one foot forward in a lunge; back leg straight. Lift the chest and bring the hands above the knee.

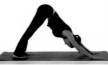

Downward Facing Dog
Straighten the legs and lift the tailbone toward the ceiling. Weight evenly distributed between hands and feet.

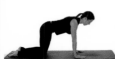

Table
Get on all fours with shoulders and knees hip distance apart. Distribute weight evenly across both hands feet.

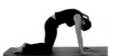

Cat Pose 2
Exhale and arch the back, tucking the chin and tailbone under.

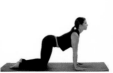

Cat Pose
Inhale and relax the belly towards the floor, lifting the head and tailbone toward the sky.

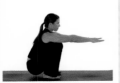

Squat
With big toes and heels touching, squat with wide knees and balance weight on the balls of the feet.

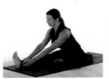

Seated Forward Bend
Sit upright with one leg extended out in front of you and the other secured against the inner thigh. Reach forward over the straight leg and grab your ankle.

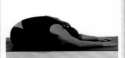

Simple Crossed Legs
Sit with legs crossed and inhale as you reach up and fold over your legs, bringing your head to the floor.

Resist-A-Ball® Workout

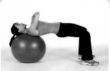

Hip Extension
Rest the head and shoulders on the ball with neck in neutral. Without moving the ball, lower and lift the hips.

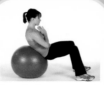

Trunk Curl
From seated position on the ball, lower down into an inclined position and curl the ribs down toward the hips.

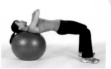

Hip Extension
Rest the head and shoulders on the ball with neck in neutral. Without moving the ball, lower and lift the hips.

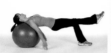

Hip Extension: One Leg Lift
Rest the head and shoulders on the ball with neck in neutral. Without moving the ball, lower and lift one leg.

Seated Walking to Seated
Begin seated on the ball. Walk the feet forward, allowing your body to roll down the ball toward the floor. Then walk the feet back to starting position.

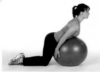

Trunk Extension
Start by placing the ball beneath your core. Press the pelvis into the ball while extending the spine away from the ball.

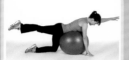

Opposition Arm/Leg
Place the ball beneath your core and kneel on all fours around the ball. Raise one leg and opposite arm. Switch.

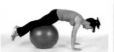

Spinal & Hip Flexion
Rest your knees on the ball with your body in push-up position. Roll your knees to pull the ball forward. Then roll back.

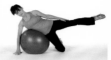

Hip Abduction
Begin kneeling and lean sideways over the ball, securing one hand on the ground. Press the hip into the ball and raise the outside leg. Lower, and repeat.

Knee Extension
Place the ball between the feet. Squeeze the legs together as you lift the ball toward the ceiling. Lower down and repeat.

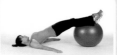

Hip Extension
Rest the head and shoulders on the floor with neck in neutral. Without moving the ball, lower and lift the hips.

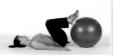

Leg Curl
Lie with your back on the floor and place your heels on the top of the ball. Push with the heels to roll the ball forward and back, While crunching the Abs.

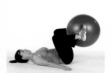

Leg Press
Lie on back with the ball elevated between the feet. Bend knees and then straighten the legs with abs contracted.

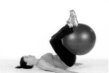

Reverse Trunk Curl
Lie on back with knees bent over the ball. Then, clamp down on the ball with legs and feet to lift the ball off the floor.

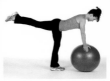

Standing Hip Extension
Place hands on top of the ball and lift one leg toward the back wall, squeezing the glutes. Switch.

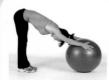

Pike Stretch
Bend at the hips and place the hands on top of the ball. Push your tailbone backward and upward while extending your arms for a stretch.

Back Stretch
Stand with feet hip-distance apart and bend the knees. Hold the ball between the arms and knees, and tuck the chin under while rounding the back.

Lateral Trunk Stretch
Place feet shoulder width apart. Hold the ball under one arm and shift your weight over the ball as you reach to the side and flex the spine.

Mat Core Challenge Workout

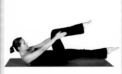

Single Leg Stretch
Lie on your mat, head lifted, abs crunched; reaching toward your bent knee. Release leg and switch.

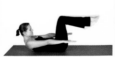

Hundred
Raise your head and legs off the floor, knees bent, and take short, rapid breaths as you pump your arms and hold the pose.

Leg Circles
Lying on the mat, extend your leg toward the ceiling and circle it across your midline and back.

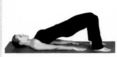

Shoulder Bridge
Inhale and lift the spine off the mat while curling the pelvis upward into a posterior tilt.

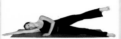

Sidelying Up/Down (right side)
Lying on your side, rest your head on your extended arm and lift the top leg up and down, keeping your hips and shoulders stacked.

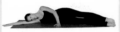

Sidelying Circles (right side)
Lying on your side, stack your hips and shoulders and lift the top leg to hip height, circling it behind and back around. Keep foot pointed.

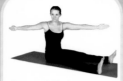

Seated Twist
Sit tall with legs extended. Inhale to prepare for the movement. Exhale and twist your spine, bringing your ribcage to the right. Repeat on left.

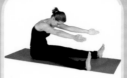

Seated Spine Stretch
Inhale and round your spine forward, reaching your arms parallel to your legs.

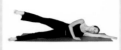

Sidelying Up/Down (left side)
Lying on your side, rest your head on your extended arm and lift the top leg up and down, keeping your hips and shoulders stacked.

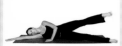

Sidelying Circles (right side)

Lying on your side, stack your hips and shoulders and lift the top leg to hip height, circling it behind and back around. Keep foot pointed.

Prone Flight

Inhale as you lift your head and upper body off the mat.
Keep the tops of your feet on the floor.

Prone Swimming

Inhale as you lift your right arm and left leg while keeping your head on the floor. Switch.

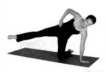

Kneeling Side Kick (right side)

From a kneeling position, inhale and bring one hand down to the mat while lifting the opposite leg to hip height.

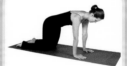

All Fours Balance

Kneel on the mat on all fours, aligning your hands underneath your shoulders and knees beneath your hips.

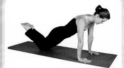

Plank (modified)

Kneel on the mat with both knees together and feet lifted. Place your hands in line with your shoulders.

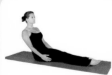

Hip Hinge Front/Back

Sit tall with your legs extended. Exhale and hinge your spine forward. Inhale to return to starting position, and then exhale and hinge your spine backward.

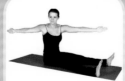

Seated Twist

Sit tall with legs extended. Inhale to prepare for the movement. Exhale and twist your spine, bringing your ribcage to the right. Repeat on left.

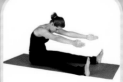

Seated Spine Stretch

Inhale and round your spine forward, reaching your arms parallel to your legs.

References:

Cunningham, Eleese, RD. "What are Interesterified Fats?" ADA Web site: http://www.eatright.org/Members/content.aspx?id=4294967578&terms=interesterified+fat

Edwards, Sally. The Heart Rate Monitor Book. Velo Press, 2000

Enig, Mary, Ph.D., and Fallon, Sally. 2003. "The Oiling of America." Health Education Alliance for Life and Longevity. (http://www.health.com/body/healthupdates/food/hydrogenatedfat.html)

Franklin J.S., B.D. Schiele, J. Brozek and A. Keys. "Observations on Human Behavior in Experimental Starvation and Rehabilitation". Journal of Clinical Psychology 4 (1948): 28-45.

Friel, Joe. The Cyclist's Training Bible. Velo Press, 2003.

G, Johnny and Kearns, Brad. The Spintensity™ Program Guide. Mad Dogg Athletics, Inc., 1999.

Keys, A., J. Brozek, A. Henschel, O. Mickelson and H.L. Taylor The Biology of Human Starvation. Minneapolis: University of Minnesota Press, 1950.

Planck, Nina. Real Food. PP. 1-4. Bloomsbury Publishing, 2006.

Polivy, Janet, Ph.D., "Psychological Consequences of Food Restriction." Journal of the American Dietetic Association 6 (1996): 589-592.

Pollan, Michael. In Defense of Food. P. 148. Penguin Press, 2008.

Riley, Gay, MS, RD, CCN. 2003. "The Marketing of Food and Diets in America" Net Nutritionist.com. (http://www.netnutritionist.com/fa.htm)

Schiele, B.C. and Brozek J. "Experimental Neurosis Resulting From Semistarvation in Man." Psychosomatic Medicine 10 (1948):31-50.

Zeman, Frances J. and Ney, Denise M. Applications in Medical Nutrition Therapy. Prentice Hall, 1995.

"Chemical Cuisine." Nutrition Action Newsletter, May 2008. http://www.cspinet.org/nah/05_08/chem_cuisine.pdf

"Hungry: Learning to Manage Your Hunger." 2003. (http://www.dietsurf.com/hungry_.htm)

"Hydrogenated Fats and Oils: Are They a Health Risk?" The Oiling of America HEALL. http://www.heall.com/body/healthupdates/food/hydrogenatedfat.html

"Obesity in America." Mayo Clinic Health.com. 2003. (http://www.cnn.com/2000/HEALTH/mayo/10/05/obesity.america/)

"The Latest Trendy Food Terms: Defined." ADA Times, Winter 2010. http://old.eatright.org/cps/rde/xchg/adatimes/hs.xsl/587.htm

SPINNING®

8-Week Weight Loss Program

Healthy Habits and
Activity Logbook

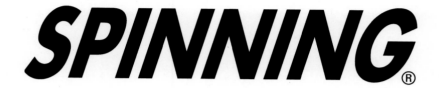

Spinning® Energy Zone™ Charts

First select the chart with the resting heart rate closest to your own. Then select the row with the AT heart rate closest to your own. That row will give you your heart rate ranges for each Energy Zone. Note: The AT heart rate matches the

RESTING HEART RATE: 50

AT Heart Rate	Recovery Energy Zone	Endurance Energy Zone	Strength Energy Zone	Intense Interval	Interval Recovery	Race Day Energy Zone
148	108-125	125-136	136-148	148-156	119	142-156
152	110-128	128-140	140-152	152-160	122	146-160
156	113-131	131-144	144-156	156-165	125	150-165
161	115-135	135-148	148-161	161-170	128	154-170
165	118-138	138-151	151-165	165-174	131	158-174
169	120-141	141-155	155-169	169-179	134	162-179
173	123-144	144-159	159-173	173-183	137	166-183
178	125-148	148-163	163-178	178-188	140	170-188
182	128-151	151-166	166-182	182-193	143	174-193
186	130-154	154-170	170-186	186-197	146	178-197

RESTING HEART RATE: 60

AT Heart Rate	Recovery Energy Zone	Endurance Energy Zone	Strength Energy Zone	Intense Interval	Interval Recovery	Race Day Energy Zone
149	113-128	128-139	139-149	149-157	123	144-157
154	115-132	132-143	143-154	154-161	126	148-161
158	118-135	135-146	146-158	158-166	129	152-166
162	120-138	138-150	150-162	162-170	132	156-170

upper end of the Strength Energy Zone. Record your heart rate zones in your logbook for easy reference. You will need to refer to these numbers each time you take part in a Spinning® ride.

RESTING HEART RATE: 70

AT Heart Rate	Recovery Energy Zone	Endurance Energy Zone	Strength Energy Zone	Intense Interval	Interval Recovery	Race Day Energy Zone
151	118-132	132-141	141-151	151-157	127	146-157
155	120-135	135-145	145-155	155-162	130	150-162
159	123-138	138-149	149-159	159-167	133	154-167
164	125-142	142-153	153-164	164-171	136	158-171
168	128-145	145-156	156-168	168-176	139	162-176
172	130-148	148-160	160-172	172-180	142	166-180
176	133-151	151-164	164-176	176-185	145	170-185
181	135-155	155-168	168-181	181-190	148	174-190
185	138-158	158-171	171-185	185-194	151	178-194
189	140-161	161-175	175-189	189-199	154	182-199

166	123-141	141-154	154-166	166-175	135	160-175
171	125-145	145-158	158-171	171-180	138	164-180
175	128-148	148-161	161-175	175-184	141	168-184
179	130-151	151-165	165-179	179-189	144	172-189
183	133-154	154-169	169-183	183-193	147	176-193
188	135-158	158-173	173-188	188-198	150	180-198

AGE BASED HEART RATE CHART

AGE	RECOVERY 50%-65%	ENDURANCE 65%-75%	STRENGTH 75%-85%	INTERVAL 65%-92%	RACE DAY 80%-92%
20-23	100-129	129-149	149-168	129-182	160-182
24-27	98-126	126-146	146-165	126-178	155-178
28-31	96-123	123-143	143-162	123-175	153-175
32-35	94-120	120-140	140-159	120-172	150-172
36-39	92-118	118-137	137-155	118-168	146-168
40-43	90-116	116-134	134-151	116-164	143-164
44-47	88-113	113-131	131-148	113-161	140-162
48-51	86-110	110-128	128-145	110-157	137-157
52-55	84-108	108-125	125-141	108-153	133-153
56-60	82-105	105-122	122-139	105-150	131-150

Example: If you're 30 years old, your target hreat rate for the Endurance Energy Zone™
is 123-143 beates per minute

Initial, Mid-Point and Final Measurements

	Initial Measurements Date:_____	4-Week Measurements Date:_____	Final Measurements Date:_____
Weight			
Circumference Measurements			
Right Upper Arm			
Left Upper Arm			
Chest			
Waist			
Hips			
Right Thigh			
Left Thigh			
Heart Rate Information			
Resting Heart Rate			
Anaerobic Threshold			
Recovery Energy Zone™			
Endurance Energy Zone™			
Strength Energy Zone™			
Interval Energy Zone™			
Interval Recovery			
Race Day Energy Zone™			
Excercise Program (circle one)	1 2 3 4	1 2 3 4	1 2 3 4

Total Weight Loss		
Total Inches Lost		
Change in Anaerobic Threshold		

	Week 1	Week 2	Week 3	Week 4	Week 5	Week 6	Week 7	Week 8
Total Healthy Habits Points								
Total Activity Minutes								

Daily Tracking Sheet

Sunday: ___*October* __12_____
             month   date

Healthy Habits	Point Value	Points Earned
1. Stayed within a 3 and a 6 on the hunger - satiety scale.	20	*20*
2. Drank at least 64 ounces of water.	30	*25*
Total Points		*45*

Activity	Recovery	Endurance	Strength	Interval	Race Day	Total Training Time
Spinning	*10*	*30*				*40*
Walking	*20*					*20*
Total Training Time	*30*	*30*				*60*

☐ Yoga Asana Sequence
☐ Resist-A-Ball®
☐ Mat Core Challenge

Total Healthy Habits Points: _____ 210 _____

Total Activity minutes: _____ 140 _____

Activity	Time spent in Energy Zone™ (minutes)					
	Recovery	Endurance	Strength	Interval	Race Day	Total Training Time
Spinning		105	15			120
Walking	20					20
% Total Training Time	15%	75%	10%			140

Notes:

_____   _____

_____

_____

_____

_____

_____

_____

_____

_____

_____

_____

Daily Tracking Sheet

Sunday: _____
                month   date

Healthy Habits	Point Value	Points Earned
1. Stayed within a 3 and a 6 on the hunger - satiety scale.	20	
2. Drank at least 64 ounces of water.	30	
Total Points:	50	

Activity	Time spent in Energy Zone™ (minutes)					
	Recovery	Endurance	Strength	Interval	Race Day	Total Training Time
Total Training Time						

☐ Yoga Asana Sequence
☐ Resist-A-Ball®
☐ Mat Core Challenge

Daily Tracking Sheet

Monday: _____
               month   date

Healthy Habits	Point Value	Points Earned
1. Stayed within a 3 and a 6 on the hunger - satiety scale.	20	
2. Drank at least 64 ounces of water.	30	
Total Points:	50	

	Time spent in Energy Zone™ (minutes)					
Activity	Recovery	Endurance	Strength	Interval	Race Day	Total Training Time
Total Training Time						

☐ Yoga Asana Sequence
☐ Resist-A-Ball®
☐ Mat Core Challenge

Daily Tracking Sheet

Tuesday: ———————————————————
month   date

Healthy Habits	Point Value	Points Earned
1. Stayed within a 3 and a 6 on the hunger - satiety scale.	20	
2. Drank at least 64 ounces of water.	30	
Total Points:	50	

	Time spent in Energy Zone™ (minutes)					
Activity	Recovery	Endurance	Strength	Interval	Race Day	Total Training Time
Total Training Time						

☐ Yoga Asana Sequence
☐ Resist-A-Ball®
☐ Mat Core Challenge

Daily Tracking Sheet

Wednesday: _____
            month   date

Healthy Habits	Point Value	Points Earned
1. Stayed within a 3 and a 6 on the hunger - satiety scale.	20	
2. Drank at least 64 ounces of water.	30	
Total Points:	50	

Activity	Time spent in Energy Zone™ (minutes)					
	Recovery	Endurance	Strength	Interval	Race Day	Total Training Time
Total Training Time						

☐ Yoga Asana Sequence
☐ Resist-A-Ball®
☐ Mat Core Challenge

Daily Tracking Sheet

Thursday: _____
        month   date

Healthy Habits	Point Value	Points Earned
1. Stayed within a 3 and a 6 on the hunger - satiety scale.	20	
2. Drank at least 64 ounces of water.	30	
Total Points:	50	

Activity	Time spent in Energy Zone™ (minutes)					
	Recovery	Endurance	Strength	Interval	Race Day	Total Training Time
Total Training Time						

☐ Yoga Asana Sequence
☐ Resist-A-Ball®
☐ Mat Core Challenge

Daily Tracking Sheet

Friday: _____
　　　　　　　month　　　　　　date

Healthy Habits	Point Value	Points Earned
1. Stayed within a 3 and a 6 on the hunger - satiety scale.	20	
2. Drank at least 64 ounces of water.	30	
Total Points:	50	

Activity	Time spent in Energy Zone™ (minutes)					
	Recovery	Endurance	Strength	Interval	Race Day	Total Training Time
Total Training Time						

☐ Yoga Asana Sequence
☐ Resist-A-Ball®
☐ Mat Core Challenge

Daily Tracking Sheet

Saturday: _____
                month   date

Healthy Habits	Point Value	Points Earned
1. Stayed within a 3 and a 6 on the hunger - satiety scale.	20	
2. Drank at least 64 ounces of water.	30	
Total Points:	50	

	Time spent in Energy Zone™ (minutes)					
Activity	Recovery	Endurance	Strength	Interval	Race Day	Total Training Time
Total Training Time						

☐ Yoga Asana Sequence
☐ Resist-A-Ball®
☐ Mat Core Challenge

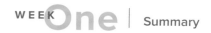

WEEK **One** | Summary

Total Healthy Habits Points: _____

Total Activity Minutes: _____

Activity	Time spent in Energy Zone™ (minutes)					Total Training Time
	Recovery	Endurance	Strength	Interval	Race Day	
% Total Training Time						

Notes:

_____

_____

_____

_____

_____

_____

_____

_____

_____

_____

_____

Daily Tracking Sheet

Sunday: _____

Healthy Habits	Point Value	Points Earned
1. Stayed within a 3 and a 6 on the hunger - satiety scale.	20	
2. Drank at least 64 ounces of water.	30	
3. Ate a healthy breakfast.	30	
4. Did not snack after dinner.	30	
Total Points:	110	

	Time spent in Energy Zone™ (minutes)					
Activity	Recovery	Endurance	Strength	Interval	Race Day	Total Training Time
Total Training Time						

☐ Yoga Asana Sequence
☐ Resist-A-Ball®
☐ Mat Core Challenge

Daily Tracking Sheet

Monday: _____
              month   date

Healthy Habits	Point Value	Points Earned
1. Stayed within a 3 and a 6 on the hunger - satiety scale.	20	
2. Drank at least 64 ounces of water.	30	
3. Ate a healthy breakfast.	30	
4. Did not snack after dinner.	30	
Total Points:	110	

	Time spent in Energy Zone™ (minutes)					
Activity	Recovery	Endurance	Strength	Interval	Race Day	Total Training Time
Total Training Time						

☐ Yoga Asana Sequence
☐ Resist-A-Ball®
☐ Mat Core Challenge

Daily Tracking Sheet

Tuesday: _____
          month   date

Healthy Habits	Point Value	Points Earned
1. Stayed within a 3 and a 6 on the hunger - satiety scale.	20	
2. Drank at least 64 ounces of water.	30	
3. Ate a healthy breakfast.	30	
4. Did not snack after dinner.	30	
Total Points:	110	

| Activity | Time spent in Energy Zone™ (minutes) | | | | | Total Training Time |
	Recovery	Endurance	Strength	Interval	Race Day	
Total Training Time						

☐ Yoga Asana Sequence
☐ Resist-A-Ball®
☐ Mat Core Challenge

Daily Tracking Sheet

Wednesday: _____
month   date

Healthy Habits	Point Value	Points Earned
1. Stayed within a 3 and a 6 on the hunger - satiety scale.	20	
2. Drank at least 64 ounces of water.	30	
3. Ate a healthy breakfast.	30	
4. Did not snack after dinner.	30	
Total Points:	110	

Activity	Time spent in Energy Zone™ (minutes)					
	Recovery	Endurance	Strength	Interval	Race Day	Total Training Time
Total Training Time						

☐ Yoga Asana Sequence
☐ Resist-A-Ball®
☐ Mat Core Challenge

Daily Tracking Sheet

Thursday: _____
   month   date

Healthy Habits	Point Value	Points Earned
1. Stayed within a 3 and a 6 on the hunger - satiety scale.	20	
2. Drank at least 64 ounces of water.	30	
3. Ate a healthy breakfast.	30	
4. Did not snack after dinner.	30	
Total Points:	110	

	Time spent in Energy Zone™ (minutes)					
Activity	Recovery	Endurance	Strength	Interval	Race Day	Total Training Time
Total Training Time						

☐ Yoga Asana Sequence
☐ Resist-A-Ball®
☐ Mat Core Challenge

Daily Tracking Sheet

Friday: _____
           month   date

Healthy Habits	Point Value	Points Earned
1. Stayed within a 3 and a 6 on the hunger - satiety scale.	20	
2. Drank at least 64 ounces of water.	30	
3. Ate a healthy breakfast.	30	
4. Did not snack after dinner.	30	
Total Points:	110	

Activity	Time spent in Energy Zone™ (minutes)					Total Training Time
	Recovery	Endurance	Strength	Interval	Race Day	
Total Training Time						

☐ Yoga Asana Sequence
☐ Resist-A-Ball®
☐ Mat Core Challenge

Daily Tracking Sheet

Saturday: _____
            month   date

Healthy Habits	Point Value	Points Earned
1. Stayed within a 3 and a 6 on the hunger - satiety scale.	20	
2. Drank at least 64 ounces of water.	30	
3. Ate a healthy breakfast.	30	
4. Did not snack after dinner.	30	
Total Points:	110	

Activity	Time spent in Energy Zone™ (minutes)					Total Training Time
	Recovery	Endurance	Strength	Interval	Race Day	
Total Training Time						

☐ Yoga Asana Sequence
☐ Resist-A-Ball®
☐ Mat Core Challenge

WEEK 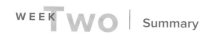 **TWO** | Summary

Total Healthy Habits Points: _____

Total Activity Minutes: _____

Activity	Time spent in Energy Zone™ (minutes)					
	Recovery	Endurance	Strength	Interval	Race Day	Total Training Time
% Total Training Time						

Notes:

_____

_____

_____

_____

_____

_____

_____

_____

_____

_____

_____

Daily Tracking Sheet

Sunday: _____
month   date

Healthy Habits	Point Value	Points Earned
1. Stayed within a 3 and a 6 on the hunger - satiety scale.	20	
2. Drank at least 64 ounces of water.	30	
3. Ate a healthy breakfast.	30	
4. Did not snack after dinner.	30	
5. Ate at least 6 fruit & vegetable servings.	30	
6. Did not eat sweets or drink any alcohol.	40	
Total Points:	180	

	Time spent in Energy Zone™ (minutes)					
Activity	Recovery	Endurance	Strength	Interval	Race Day	Total Training Time
Total Training Time						

☐ Yoga Asana Sequence
☐ Resist-A-Ball®
☐ Mat Core Challenge

Daily Tracking Sheet

Monday: _____
  month   date

Healthy Habits	Point Value	Points Earned
1. Stayed within a 3 and a 6 on the hunger - satiety scale.	20	
2. Drank at least 64 ounces of water.	30	
3. Ate a healthy breakfast.	30	
4. Did not snack after dinner.	30	
5. Ate at least 6 fruit & vegetable servings.	30	
6. Did not eat sweets or drink any alcohol.	40	
Total Points:	180	

Activity	Time spent in Energy Zone™ (minutes)					
	Recovery	Endurance	Strength	Interval	Race Day	Total Training Time
Total Training Time						

☐ Yoga Asana Sequence
☐ Resist-A-Ball®
☐ Mat Core Challenge

Daily Tracking Sheet

Tuesday: _____
    month   date

Healthy Habits	Point Value	Points Earned
1. Stayed within a 3 and a 6 on the hunger - satiety scale.	20	
2. Drank at least 64 ounces of water.	30	
3. Ate a healthy breakfast.	30	
4. Did not snack after dinner.	30	
5. Ate at least 6 fruit & vegetable servings.	30	
6. Did not eat sweets or drink any alcohol.	40	
Total Points:	180	

	Time spent in Energy Zone™ (minutes)					
Activity	Recovery	Endurance	Strength	Interval	Race Day	Total Training Time
Total Training Time						

☐ Yoga Asana Sequence
☐ Resist-A-Ball®
☐ Mat Core Challenge

Daily Tracking Sheet

Wednesday: _____
            month   date

Healthy Habits	Point Value	Points Earned
1. Stayed within a 3 and a 6 on the hunger - satiety scale.	20	
2. Drank at least 64 ounces of water.	30	
3. Ate a healthy breakfast.	30	
4. Did not snack after dinner.	30	
5. Ate at least 6 fruit & vegetable servings.	30	
6. Did not eat sweets or drink any alcohol.	40	
Total Points:	180	

Activity	Time spent in Energy Zone™ (minutes)					
	Recovery	Endurance	Strength	Interval	Race Day	Total Training Time
Total Training Time						

☐ Yoga Asana Sequence
☐ Resist-A-Ball®
☐ Mat Core Challenge

Daily Tracking Sheet

Thursday: _____
month   date

Healthy Habits	Point Value	Points Earned
1. Stayed within a 3 and a 6 on the hunger - satiety scale.	20	
2. Drank at least 64 ounces of water.	30	
3. Ate a healthy breakfast.	30	
4. Did not snack after dinner.	30	
5. Ate at least 6 fruit & vegetable servings.	30	
6. Did not eat sweets or drink any alcohol.	40	
Total Points:	180	

	Time spent in Energy Zone™ (minutes)					
Activity	Recovery	Endurance	Strength	Interval	Race Day	Total Training Time
Total Training Time						

☐ Yoga Asana Sequence
☐ Resist-A-Ball®
☐ Mat Core Challenge

Daily Tracking Sheet

Friday: _____
 month   date

Healthy Habits	Point Value	Points Earned
1. Stayed within a 3 and a 6 on the hunger - satiety scale.	20	
2. Drank at least 64 ounces of water.	30	
3. Ate a healthy breakfast.	30	
4. Did not snack after dinner.	30	
5. Ate at least 6 fruit & vegetable servings.	30	
6. Did not eat sweets or drink any alcohol.	40	
Total Points:	180	

Activity	Time spent in Energy Zone™ (minutes)					
	Recovery	Endurance	Strength	Interval	Race Day	Total Training Time
Total Training Time						

☐ Yoga Asana Sequence
☐ Resist-A-Ball®
☐ Mat Core Challenge

Daily Tracking Sheet

Saturday: _____
month   date

Healthy Habits	Point Value	Points Earned
1. Stayed within a 3 and a 6 on the hunger - satiety scale.	20	
2. Drank at least 64 ounces of water.	30	
3. Ate a healthy breakfast.	30	
4. Did not snack after dinner.	30	
5. Ate at least 6 fruit & vegetable servings.	30	
6. Did not eat sweets or drink any alcohol.	40	
Total Points:	180	

	Time spent in Energy Zone™ (minutes)					
Activity	Recovery	Endurance	Strength	Interval	Race Day	Total Training Time
Total Training Time						

☐ Yoga Asana Sequence
☐ Resist-A-Ball®
☐ Mat Core Challenge

WEEK Three | Summary

Total Healthy Habits Points: _____

Total Activity Minutes: _____

Activity	Time spent in Energy Zone™ (minutes)					
	Recovery	Endurance	Strength	Interval	Race Day	Total Training Time
% Total Training Time						

Notes:

_____

_____

_____

_____

_____

_____

_____

_____

_____

_____

_____

Daily Tracking Sheet

Sunday: _____
　　　　　　month　　　　date

Healthy Habits	Point Value	Points Earned
1. Stayed within a 3 and a 6 on the hunger - satiety scale.	20	
2. Drank at least 64 ounces of water.	30	
3. Ate a healthy breakfast.	30	
4. Did not snack after dinner.	30	
5. Ate at least 6 fruit & vegetable servings.	30	
6. Did not eat sweets or drink any alcohol.	40	
7. Did not consume any hydrogenated fats.	40	
8. Did not add excess fats to foods.	20	
Total Points:	240	

Activity	Time spent in Energy Zone™ (minutes)					
	Recovery	Endurance	Strength	Interval	Race Day	Total Training Time
Total Training Time						

☐ Yoga Asana Sequence
☐ Resist-A-Ball®
☐ Mat Core Challenge

Daily Tracking Sheet

Monday: _____
            month   date

Healthy Habits	Point Value	Points Earned
1. Stayed within a 3 and a 6 on the hunger - satiety scale.	20	
2. Drank at least 64 ounces of water.	30	
3. Ate a healthy breakfast.	30	
4. Did not snack after dinner.	30	
5. Ate at least 6 fruit & vegetable servings.	30	
6. Did not eat sweets or drink any alcohol.	40	
7. Did not consume any hydrogenated fats.	40	
8. Did not add excess fats to foods.	20	
Total Points:	240	

	Time spent in Energy Zone™ (minutes)					
Activity	Recovery	Endurance	Strength	Interval	Race Day	Total Training Time
Total Training Time						

☐ Yoga Asana Sequence
☐ Resist-A-Ball®
☐ Mat Core Challenge

Daily Tracking Sheet

Tuesday: _____
          month   date

Healthy Habits	Point Value	Points Earned
1. Stayed within a 3 and a 6 on the hunger - satiety scale.	20	
2. Drank at least 64 ounces of water.	30	
3. Ate a healthy breakfast.	30	
4. Did not snack after dinner.	30	
5. Ate at least 6 fruit & vegetable servings.	30	
6. Did not eat sweets or drink any alcohol.	40	
7. Did not consume any hydrogenated fats.	40	
8. Did not add excess fats to foods.	20	
Total Points:	240	

	Time spent in Energy Zone™ (minutes)					
Activity	Recovery	Endurance	Strength	Interval	Race Day	Total Training Time
Total Training Time						

☐ Yoga Asana Sequence
☐ Resist-A-Ball®
☐ Mat Core Challenge

Daily Tracking Sheet

Wednesday: _____
month   date

Healthy Habits	Point Value	Points Earned
1. Stayed within a 3 and a 6 on the hunger - satiety scale.	20	
2. Drank at least 64 ounces of water.	30	
3. Ate a healthy breakfast.	30	
4. Did not snack after dinner.	30	
5. Ate at least 6 fruit & vegetable servings.	30	
6. Did not eat sweets or drink any alcohol.	40	
7. Did not consume any hydrogenated fats.	40	
8. Did not add excess fats to foods.	20	
Total Points:	240	

	Time spent in Energy Zone™ (minutes)					
Activity	Recovery	Endurance	Strength	Interval	Race Day	Total Training Time
Total Training Time						

☐ Yoga Asana Sequence
☐ Resist-A-Ball®
☐ Mat Core Challenge

Daily Tracking Sheet

Thursday: _____
month   date

Healthy Habits	Point Value	Points Earned
1. Stayed within a 3 and a 6 on the hunger - satiety scale.	20	
2. Drank at least 64 ounces of water.	30	
3. Ate a healthy breakfast.	30	
4. Did not snack after dinner.	30	
5. Ate at least 6 fruit & vegetable servings.	30	
6. Did not eat sweets or drink any alcohol.	40	
7. Did not consume any hydrogenated fats.	40	
8. Did not add excess fats to foods.	20	
Total Points:	240	

	Time spent in Energy Zone™ (minutes)					
Activity	Recovery	Endurance	Strength	Interval	Race Day	Total Training Time
Total Training Time						

☐ Yoga Asana Sequence
☐ Resist-A-Ball®
☐ Mat Core Challenge

Daily Tracking Sheet

Friday: _____
           month   date

Healthy Habits	Point Value	Points Earned
1. Stayed within a 3 and a 6 on the hunger - satiety scale.	20	
2. Drank at least 64 ounces of water.	30	
3. Ate a healthy breakfast.	30	
4. Did not snack after dinner.	30	
5. Ate at least 6 fruit & vegetable servings.	30	
6. Did not eat sweets or drink any alcohol.	40	
7. Did not consume any hydrogenated fats.	40	
8. Did not add excess fats to foods.	20	
Total Points:	240	

Activity	Time spent in Energy Zone™ (minutes)					
	Recovery	Endurance	Strength	Interval	Race Day	Total Training Time
Total Training Time						

☐ Yoga Asana Sequence
☐ Resist-A-Ball®
☐ Mat Core Challenge

Daily Tracking Sheet

Saturday: _____
            month   date

Healthy Habits	Point Value	Points Earned
1. Stayed within a 3 and a 6 on the hunger - satiety scale.	20	
2. Drank at least 64 ounces of water.	30	
3. Ate a healthy breakfast.	30	
4. Did not snack after dinner.	30	
5. Ate at least 6 fruit & vegetable servings.	30	
6. Did not eat sweets or drink any alcohol.	40	
7. Did not consume any hydrogenated fats.	40	
8. Did not add excess fats to foods.	20	
Total Points:	240	

Activity	Time spent in Energy Zone™ (minutes)					
	Recovery	Endurance	Strength	Interval	Race Day	Total Training Time
Total Training Time						

☐ Yoga Asana Sequence
☐ Resist-A-Ball®
☐ Mat Core Challenge

Total Healthy Habits Points: _____

Total Activity Minutes: _____

Activity	Time spent in Energy Zone™ (minutes)					
	Recovery	Endurance	Strength	Interval	Race Day	Total Training Time
% Total Training Time						

Notes:

_____

_____

_____

_____

_____

_____

_____

_____

_____

_____

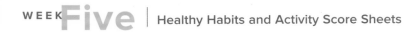
Daily Tracking Sheet

Sunday: _____
            month   date

Healthy Habits	Point Value	Points Earned
1. Stayed within a 3 and a 6 on the hunger - satiety scale.	20	
2. Drank at least 64 ounces of water.	30	
3. Ate a healthy breakfast.	30	
4. Did not snack after dinner.	30	
5. Ate at least 6 fruit & vegetable servings.	30	
6. Did not eat sweets or drink any alcohol.	40	
7. Did not consume any hydrogenated fats.	40	
8. Did not add excess fats to foods.	20	
Total Points:	240	

Activity	Time spent in Energy Zone™ (minutes)					
	Recovery	Endurance	Strength	Interval	Race Day	Total Training Time
Total Training Time						

☐ Yoga Asana Sequence
☐ Resist-A-Ball®
☐ Mat Core Challenge

Daily Tracking Sheet

Monday: _____
                 month   date

Healthy Habits	Point Value	Points Earned
1. Stayed within a 3 and a 6 on the hunger - satiety scale.	20	
2. Drank at least 64 ounces of water.	30	
3. Ate a healthy breakfast.	30	
4. Did not snack after dinner.	30	
5. Ate at least 6 fruit & vegetable servings.	30	
6. Did not eat sweets or drink any alcohol.	40	
7. Did not consume any hydrogenated fats.	40	
8. Did not add excess fats to foods.	20	
Total Points:	240	

Activity	Time spent in Energy Zone™ (minutes)					
	Recovery	Endurance	Strength	Interval	Race Day	Total Training Time
Total Training Time						

☐ Yoga Asana Sequence
☐ Resist-A-Ball®
☐ Mat Core Challenge

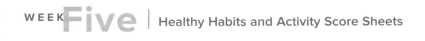

WEEK Five | Healthy Habits and Activity Score Sheets

Daily Tracking Sheet

Tuesday: _____
 month   date

Healthy Habits	Point Value	Points Earned
1. Stayed within a 3 and a 6 on the hunger - satiety scale.	20	
2. Drank at least 64 ounces of water.	30	
3. Ate a healthy breakfast.	30	
4. Did not snack after dinner.	30	
5. Ate at least 6 fruit & vegetable servings.	30	
6. Did not eat sweets or drink any alcohol.	40	
7. Did not consume any hydrogenated fats.	40	
8. Did not add excess fats to foods.	20	
Total Points:	240	

Activity	Time spent in Energy Zone™ (minutes)					
	Recovery	Endurance	Strength	Interval	Race Day	Total Training Time
Total Training Time						

☐ Yoga Asana Sequence
☐ Resist-A-Ball®
☐ Mat Core Challenge

Daily Tracking Sheet

Wednesday: _____
        month   date

Healthy Habits	Point Value	Points Earned
1. Stayed within a 3 and a 6 on the hunger - satiety scale.	20	
2. Drank at least 64 ounces of water.	30	
3. Ate a healthy breakfast.	30	
4. Did not snack after dinner.	30	
5. Ate at least 6 fruit & vegetable servings.	30	
6. Did not eat sweets or drink any alcohol.	40	
7. Did not consume any hydrogenated fats.	40	
8. Did not add excess fats to foods.	20	
Total Points:	240	

	Time spent in Energy Zone™ (minutes)					
Activity	Recovery	Endurance	Strength	Interval	Race Day	Total Training Time
Total Training Time						

☐ Yoga Asana Sequence
☐ Resist-A-Ball®
☐ Mat Core Challenge

Daily Tracking Sheet

Thursday: _____
month   date

Healthy Habits	Point Value	Points Earned
1. Stayed within a 3 and a 6 on the hunger - satiety scale.	20	
2. Drank at least 64 ounces of water.	30	
3. Ate a healthy breakfast.	30	
4. Did not snack after dinner.	30	
5. Ate at least 6 fruit & vegetable servings.	30	
6. Did not eat sweets or drink any alcohol.	40	
7. Did not consume any hydrogenated fats.	40	
8. Did not add excess fats to foods.	20	
Total Points:	240	

Activity	Time spent in Energy Zone™ (minutes)					
	Recovery	Endurance	Strength	Interval	Race Day	Total Training Time
Total Training Time						

☐ Yoga Asana Sequence
☐ Resist-A-Ball®
☐ Mat Core Challenge

Daily Tracking Sheet

Friday: _____
           month   date

Healthy Habits	Point Value	Points Earned
1. Stayed within a 3 and a 6 on the hunger - satiety scale.	20	
2. Drank at least 64 ounces of water.	30	
3. Ate a healthy breakfast.	30	
4. Did not snack after dinner.	30	
5. Ate at least 6 fruit & vegetable servings.	30	
6. Did not eat sweets or drink any alcohol.	40	
7. Did not consume any hydrogenated fats.	40	
8. Did not add excess fats to foods.	20	
Total Points:	240	

Activity	Time spent in Energy Zone™ (minutes)					
	Recovery	Endurance	Strength	Interval	Race Day	Total Training Time
Total Training Time						

☐ Yoga Asana Sequence
☐ Resist-A-Ball®
☐ Mat Core Challenge

Daily Tracking Sheet

Saturday: _____
                month   date

Healthy Habits	Point Value	Points Earned
1. Stayed within a 3 and a 6 on the hunger - satiety scale.	20	
2. Drank at least 64 ounces of water.	30	
3. Ate a healthy breakfast.	30	
4. Did not snack after dinner.	30	
5. Ate at least 6 fruit & vegetable servings.	30	
6. Did not eat sweets or drink any alcohol.	40	
7. Did not consume any hydrogenated fats.	40	
8. Did not add excess fats to foods.	20	
Total Points:	240	

	Time spent in Energy Zone™ (minutes)					
Activity	Recovery	Endurance	Strength	Interval	Race Day	Total Training Time
Total Training Time						

☐ Yoga Asana Sequence
☐ Resist-A-Ball®
☐ Mat Core Challenge

WEEK 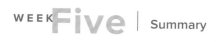 | Summary

Total Healthy Habits Points: _____

Total Activity Minutes: _____

Activity	Time spent in Energy Zone™ (minutes)					
	Recovery	Endurance	Strength	Interval	Race Day	Total Training Time
% Total Training Time						

Notes:

_____

_____

_____

_____

_____

_____

_____

_____

_____

_____

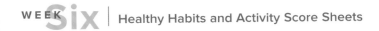

Daily Tracking Sheet

Sunday: _____
                month   date

Healthy Habits	Point Value	Points Earned
1. Stayed within a 3 and a 6 on the hunger - satiety scale.	20	
2. Drank at least 64 ounces of water.	30	
3. Ate a healthy breakfast.	30	
4. Did not snack after dinner.	30	
5. Ate at least 6 fruit & vegetable servings.	30	
6. Did not eat sweets or drink any alcohol.	40	
7. Did not consume any hydrogenated fats.	40	
8. Did not add excess fats to foods.	20	
Total Points:	240	

	Time spent in Energy Zone™ (minutes)					
Activity	Recovery	Endurance	Strength	Interval	Race Day	Total Training Time
Total Training Time						

☐ Yoga Asana Sequence
☐ Resist-A-Ball®
☐ Mat Core Challenge

Daily Tracking Sheet

Monday: _____

　　　　　month　　　　　date

Healthy Habits	Point Value	Points Earned
1. Stayed within a 3 and a 6 on the hunger - satiety scale.	20	
2. Drank at least 64 ounces of water.	30	
3. Ate a healthy breakfast.	30	
4. Did not snack after dinner.	30	
5. Ate at least 6 fruit & vegetable servings.	30	
6. Did not eat sweets or drink any alcohol.	40	
7. Did not consume any hydrogenated fats.	40	
8. Did not add excess fats to foods.	20	
Total Points:	240	

Activity	Time spent in Energy Zone™ (minutes)					
	Recovery	Endurance	Strength	Interval	Race Day	Total Training Time
Total Training Time						

☐ Yoga Asana Sequence
☐ Resist-A-Ball®
☐ Mat Core Challenge

Daily Tracking Sheet

Tuesday: _____
　　　　　　month　　　　　date

Healthy Habits	Point Value	Points Earned
1. Stayed within a 3 and a 6 on the hunger - satiety scale.	20	
2. Drank at least 64 ounces of water.	30	
3. Ate a healthy breakfast.	30	
4. Did not snack after dinner.	30	
5. Ate at least 6 fruit & vegetable servings.	30	
6. Did not eat sweets or drink any alcohol.	40	
7. Did not consume any hydrogenated fats.	40	
8. Did not add excess fats to foods.	20	
Total Points:	240	

	Time spent in Energy Zone™ (minutes)					
Activity	Recovery	Endurance	Strength	Interval	Race Day	Total Training Time
Total Training Time						

☐ Yoga Asana Sequence
☐ Resist-A-Ball®
☐ Mat Core Challenge

Daily Tracking Sheet

Wednesday: _____
                    month   date

Healthy Habits	Point Value	Points Earned
1. Stayed within a 3 and a 6 on the hunger - satiety scale.	20	
2. Drank at least 64 ounces of water.	30	
3. Ate a healthy breakfast.	30	
4. Did not snack after dinner.	30	
5. Ate at least 6 fruit & vegetable servings.	30	
6. Did not eat sweets or drink any alcohol.	40	
7. Did not consume any hydrogenated fats.	40	
8. Did not add excess fats to foods.	20	
Total Points:	240	

Activity	Time spent in Energy Zone™ (minutes)					
	Recovery	Endurance	Strength	Interval	Race Day	Total Training Time
Total Training Time						

☐ Yoga Asana Sequence
☐ Resist-A-Ball®
☐ Mat Core Challenge

Daily Tracking Sheet

Thursday: _____
                month   date

Healthy Habits	Point Value	Points Earned
1. Stayed within a 3 and a 6 on the hunger - satiety scale.	20	
2. Drank at least 64 ounces of water.	30	
3. Ate a healthy breakfast.	30	
4. Did not snack after dinner.	30	
5. Ate at least 6 fruit & vegetable servings.	30	
6. Did not eat sweets or drink any alcohol.	40	
7. Did not consume any hydrogenated fats.	40	
8. Did not add excess fats to foods.	20	
Total Points:	240	

Activity	Time spent in Energy Zone™ (minutes)					
	Recovery	Endurance	Strength	Interval	Race Day	Total Training Time
Total Training Time						

☐ Yoga Asana Sequence
☐ Resist-A-Ball®
☐ Mat Core Challenge

Daily Tracking Sheet

Friday: _____
　　　　　month　　　　date

Healthy Habits	Point Value	Points Earned
1. Stayed within a 3 and a 6 on the hunger - satiety scale.	20	
2. Drank at least 64 ounces of water.	30	
3. Ate a healthy breakfast.	30	
4. Did not snack after dinner.	30	
5. Ate at least 6 fruit & vegetable servings.	30	
6. Did not eat sweets or drink any alcohol.	40	
7. Did not consume any hydrogenated fats.	40	
8. Did not add excess fats to foods.	20	
Total Points:	240	

	Time spent in Energy Zone™ (minutes)					
Activity	Recovery	Endurance	Strength	Interval	Race Day	Total Training Time
Total Training Time						

☐ Yoga Asana Sequence
☐ Resist-A-Ball®
☐ Mat Core Challenge

Daily Tracking Sheet

Saturday: _____
          month   date

Healthy Habits	Point Value	Points Earned
1. Stayed within a 3 and a 6 on the hunger - satiety scale.	20	
2. Drank at least 64 ounces of water.	30	
3. Ate a healthy breakfast.	30	
4. Did not snack after dinner.	30	
5. Ate at least 6 fruit & vegetable servings.	30	
6. Did not eat sweets or drink any alcohol.	40	
7. Did not consume any hydrogenated fats.	40	
8. Did not add excess fats to foods.	20	
Total Points:	240	

	Time spent in Energy Zone™ (minutes)					
Activity	Recovery	Endurance	Strength	Interval	Race Day	Total Training Time
Total Training Time						

☐ Yoga Asana Sequence
☐ Resist-A-Ball®
☐ Mat Core Challenge

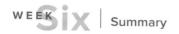

WEEK **Six** | Summary

Total Healthy Habits Points: _____

Total Activity Minutes: _____

Activity	Time spent in Energy Zone™ (minutes)					
	Recovery	Endurance	Strength	Interval	Race Day	Total Training Time
% Total Training Time						

Notes:

_____

_____

_____

_____

_____

_____

_____

_____

_____

_____

Daily Tracking Sheet

Sunday: _____
            month   date

Healthy Habits	Point Value	Points Earned
1. Stayed within a 3 and a 6 on the hunger - satiety scale.	20	
2. Drank at least 64 ounces of water.	30	
3. Ate a healthy breakfast.	30	
4. Did not snack after dinner.	30	
5. Ate at least 6 fruit & vegetable servings.	30	
6. Did not eat sweets or drink any alcohol.	40	
7. Did not consume any hydrogenated fats.	40	
8. Did not add excess fats to foods.	20	
Total Points:	240	

Activity	Time spent in Energy Zone™ (minutes)					
	Recovery	Endurance	Strength	Interval	Race Day	Total Training Time
Total Training Time						

☐ Yoga Asana Sequence
☐ Resist-A-Ball®
☐ Mat Core Challenge

Daily Tracking Sheet

Monday: _____
          month   date

Healthy Habits	Point Value	Points Earned
1. Stayed within a 3 and a 6 on the hunger - satiety scale.	20	
2. Drank at least 64 ounces of water.	30	
3. Ate a healthy breakfast.	30	
4. Did not snack after dinner.	30	
5. Ate at least 6 fruit & vegetable servings.	30	
6. Did not eat sweets or drink any alcohol.	40	
7. Did not consume any hydrogenated fats.	40	
8. Did not add excess fats to foods.	20	
Total Points:	240	

Activity	Time spent in Energy Zone™ (minutes)					
	Recovery	Endurance	Strength	Interval	Race Day	Total Training Time
Total Training Time						

☐ Yoga Asana Sequence
☐ Resist-A-Ball®
☐ Mat Core Challenge

Daily Tracking Sheet

Tuesday: _____
　　　　　　　month　　　　　　date

Healthy Habits	Point Value	Points Earned
1. Stayed within a 3 and a 6 on the hunger - satiety scale.	20	
2. Drank at least 64 ounces of water.	30	
3. Ate a healthy breakfast.	30	
4. Did not snack after dinner.	30	
5. Ate at least 6 fruit & vegetable servings.	30	
6. Did not eat sweets or drink any alcohol.	40	
7. Did not consume any hydrogenated fats.	40	
8. Did not add excess fats to foods.	20	
Total Points:	240	

	Time spent in Energy Zone™ (minutes)					
Activity	Recovery	Endurance	Strength	Interval	Race Day	Total Training Time
Total Training Time						

☐ Yoga Asana Sequence
☐ Resist-A-Ball®
☐ Mat Core Challenge

Daily Tracking Sheet

Wednesday: _____
 month   date

Healthy Habits	Point Value	Points Earned
1. Stayed within a 3 and a 6 on the hunger - satiety scale.	20	
2. Drank at least 64 ounces of water.	30	
3. Ate a healthy breakfast.	30	
4. Did not snack after dinner.	30	
5. Ate at least 6 fruit & vegetable servings.	30	
6. Did not eat sweets or drink any alcohol.	40	
7. Did not consume any hydrogenated fats.	40	
8. Did not add excess fats to foods.	20	
Total Points:	240	

Activity	Time spent in Energy Zone™ (minutes)					
	Recovery	Endurance	Strength	Interval	Race Day	Total Training Time
Total Training Time						

☐ Yoga Asana Sequence
☐ Resist-A-Ball®
☐ Mat Core Challenge

Daily Tracking Sheet

Thursday: _____
            month   date

Healthy Habits	Point Value	Points Earned
1. Stayed within a 3 and a 6 on the hunger - satiety scale.	20	
2. Drank at least 64 ounces of water.	30	
3. Ate a healthy breakfast.	30	
4. Did not snack after dinner.	30	
5. Ate at least 6 fruit & vegetable servings.	30	
6. Did not eat sweets or drink any alcohol.	40	
7. Did not consume any hydrogenated fats.	40	
8. Did not add excess fats to foods.	20	
Total Points:	240	

	Time spent in Energy Zone™ (minutes)					
Activity	Recovery	Endurance	Strength	Interval	Race Day	Total Training Time
Total Training Time						

☐ Yoga Asana Sequence
☐ Resist-A-Ball®
☐ Mat Core Challenge

Daily Tracking Sheet

Friday: _____
        month   date

Healthy Habits	Point Value	Points Earned
1. Stayed within a 3 and a 6 on the hunger - satiety scale.	20	
2. Drank at least 64 ounces of water.	30	
3. Ate a healthy breakfast.	30	
4. Did not snack after dinner.	30	
5. Ate at least 6 fruit & vegetable servings.	30	
6. Did not eat sweets or drink any alcohol.	40	
7. Did not consume any hydrogenated fats.	40	
8. Did not add excess fats to foods.	20	
Total Points:	240	

Activity	Time spent in Energy Zone™ (minutes)					
	Recovery	Endurance	Strength	Interval	Race Day	Total Training Time
Total Training Time						

☐ Yoga Asana Sequence
☐ Resist-A-Ball®
☐ Mat Core Challenge

Daily Tracking Sheet

Saturday: _____
month   date

Healthy Habits	Point Value	Points Earned
1. Stayed within a 3 and a 6 on the hunger - satiety scale.	20	
2. Drank at least 64 ounces of water.	30	
3. Ate a healthy breakfast.	30	
4. Did not snack after dinner.	30	
5. Ate at least 6 fruit & vegetable servings.	30	
6. Did not eat sweets or drink any alcohol.	40	
7. Did not consume any hydrogenated fats.	40	
8. Did not add excess fats to foods.	20	
Total Points:	240	

Activity	Time spent in Energy Zone™ (minutes)					
	Recovery	Endurance	Strength	Interval	Race Day	Total Training Time
Total Training Time						

☐ Yoga Asana Sequence
☐ Resist-A-Ball®
☐ Mat Core Challenge

WEEK Seven | Summary

Total Healthy Habits Points: _____

Total Activity Minutes: _____

Activity	Time spent in Energy Zone™ (minutes)					
	Recovery	Endurance	Strength	Interval	Race Day	Total Training Time
% Total Training Time						

Notes:

_____

_____

_____

_____

_____

_____

_____

_____

_____

_____

Daily Tracking Sheet

Sunday: _____
            month   date

Healthy Habits	Point Value	Points Earned
1. Stayed within a 3 and a 6 on the hunger - satiety scale.	20	
2. Drank at least 64 ounces of water.	30	
3. Ate a healthy breakfast.	30	
4. Did not snack after dinner.	30	
5. Ate at least 6 fruit & vegetable servings.	30	
6. Did not eat sweets or drink any alcohol.	40	
7. Did not consume any hydrogenated fats.	40	
8. Did not add excess fats to foods.	20	
Total Points:	240	

Activity	Time spent in Energy Zone™ (minutes)					
	Recovery	Endurance	Strength	Interval	Race Day	Total Training Time
Total Training Time						

☐ Yoga Asana Sequence
☐ Resist-A-Ball®
☐ Mat Core Challenge